6-30-70

Your Heart
Is Stronger
Than You Think

Your Heart
Is Stronger
Than You Think

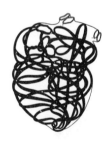

PETER J. STEINCROHN, M.D.

COWLES BOOK COMPANY, INC.
NEW YORK

1536939

In memory of Dwight D. Eisenhower,
who exemplified by his own courageous
experience in overcoming a series of
heart attacks that
YOUR HEART IS STRONGER THAN YOU THINK

"*Anxiety about the heart can be, and often is, just as harmful as heart disease.*"

—*H. M. Marvin, M.D.*

"Peace of mind *and* peace of soul—*you can have neither without* peace of heart. *Only a saint can be oblivious to heart trouble of any kind—whether it be real or imaginary. No man can be happy with a good heart if he is convinced that he has a bad heart.*"

—*Peter J. Steincrohn, M.D.*

"*Every heart specialist worth his salt must know how to take good care of the patient without heart disease who is sure he has it.*"

—*W. J. Mayo, M.D.*

"*To become an invalid without having the disease is almost as serious as to become one with it. In both situations the person is incapacitated.*"

—*Samuel Karelitz, M.D.*

CONTENTS

PART III

SPECIFIC ADVICE
FOR THE HEART–SICK

PART IV

LIVE HAPPILY
A LONG TIME AFTER

PREFACE

Maybe your heart trouble isn't real. Maybe your heart is stronger than you think.

Before you accuse me of raising false hopes, remember that this book is predicated on my more than twenty-five years' experience as an internist and cardiologist, treating thousands of heart patients at home, in my office, and at the hospital bedside.

I have come to this conclusion: People with imaginary heart trouble often suffer more than those who have actual heart disease. A fair estimate is that three out of four patients who *think* they have heart disease have normal hearts. (Instead, they suffer from heart *trouble*—not from heart disease.)

An article in *Newsweek* (Sept. 18, 1967) brings home this point quite forcefully:

> Heart disease is a real enough killer, taking some 550,000 lives a year. But it may also be one of the great neurotic ailments of all time. As many as 20 million Americans, a New York rehabilitation expert told the American Psychological Association last week, are the victims of wholly imaginary cardiac disorders.

"All of these people," said Dr. Frederick A. White-house of Hofstra University, "are living limited and anxious lives which not only affect them but their families."

Whitehouse added: "Their heart trouble may be the result of a physician's misdiagnosis or their own desire to escape responsibility."

Late one night the clatter of the telephone bell suddenly shattered the stillness and quickly disrupted my sleep. As I fumbled for the receiver, the hands of my bedside clock registered 2:30 A.M.

"Doctor," shouted an excited voice, "please come quick. My husband's having a heart attack."

Hurriedly dressing, I got into my car and drove to the address the hysterical woman gave to me. When I reached the house a few miles away, I found the patient sitting up in bed, two hamlike fists clutching at the left side of his chest. The man was a giant, dark-haired and ruddy-skinned but frightened as a small boy.

"It must be my heart," he said. "It suddenly stops and misses a beat every once in a while. Woke me right out of my sleep. At times it seems the next beat will never come. Am I dying?" There was sheer panic in his gruff, trembling voice.

The stethoscope told the story. This healthy twenty-five-year old steel worker was having harmless "heart skips." (The technical term is "premature contractions" or "extrasystoles.")

I tried to reassure him and gave him a sedative. Within the hour, as I sat at his bedside, he was deep in sleep.

This man, subsequently my patient for more than twenty-six years, never again had a similar attack of acute anxiety, although he was still susceptible to occasional recurrences of irregular heart beat. He was able to return to his precarious work on steel girders many stories above the street. He was one of the fortunate ones able to "forget about his heart."

Unlike him, many millions in the United States continue to suffer from imaginary heart trouble. (You will note I call it "trouble" and not "disease." The distinction between the two is important.)

If you live in abnormal heart fear rather than in normal heart awareness, what you must overcome is *Thanatophobia*—the fear of death. Most people will not admit it, but this is the root of their anxiety. It may become so complicated that the anxiety-ridden cardiophobe soon begins to suffer from *Phobophobia*—the fear of one's own fears. Anxiety compounds anxiety.

I have observed it again and again. Many patients actually live in constant daily apprehension. I agree with Dr. Louis A. Selverstone of Tufts University and New England Center Hospital who said, "In many people, worry and fear concerning the diagnosis of heart trouble may produce more disability than the disease itself."

Here, for example, is the case of Joe Martin, another young man with a troubled heart and mind. While he was lying quietly in bed one night, reading, his heart suddenly skipped a beat or two. Since his wife was asleep he did not wake her. This two-hundred-pound, former football tackle suddenly became transformed into a frightened, anxiety-bedeviled semi-invalid.

After a few days of silent suffering and loss of efficiency as a salesman in an appliance store, he at last communicated his fears to his wife. She insisted he see the family doctor.

Medical examination revealed a normal heart. Financial

worries, oversmoking, and gulping at least a dozen cups of coffee a day had combined to lay the groundwork for a fractious heart. Not until Joe faced his neurosis honestly did he begin to improve.

He changed his job to one he liked better and increased his income by at least fifty percent. He cut his coffee intake to one cup a day and gave up smoking. Ask him about his heart now and he will say that it isn't skittish any more.

"Most of the time it runs as smooth as a new motor," he states with a broad grin. "It only skips once in a while —and I forget it."

For centuries the heart has been the traditional center of our emotions. It has been linked with expressions of love, hate, courage, cowardice, and other evidences of human reaction to environment.

Unfortunately, we cannot change your heredity. But thankfully, we can often improve your present environment and so reshape your cardiac awareness that it is accepted as a natural phenomenon rather than a threat of extinction.

Psychosomatics is more than a fancy word. Your psyche (mind) and soma (body) are inevitably bound up together. One depends upon the other for fulfillment of its proper functions. When the normal heart is in dysfunction we look to the mind.

I never say to a patient, "Stop worrying." Worry is not like water that can be abruptly turned off as it runs through a faucet. Anxiety runs through the mind night and day. I can teach you to worry less but not how to stop worrying altogether.

The basic secret in relieving your apprehensions if you are abnormally heart-conscious is to set enough time aside to be able to "ventilate" your feelings. This is a psychiatric term which means "getting it (whatever it is) off one's chest."

Contrary to what I may imply, it doesn't suggest that I recommend that every scared heart patient lie on a couch to unburden his mind. You can do as well in your doctor's office, sitting in a chair.

What is essential, though, is that your doctor be a sympathetic, humane listener. If the doctor's eyes are on the hands of the clock during the interview, failure is the usual result. The patient with imaginary heart trouble continues to believe that he has heart disease.

In these busy days a shortage of physicians necessarily places a premium on time; it is my purpose in this book to help take up the slack. To be an intermediate "listening post." And to give you practical advice on ridding yourself of unnatural anxiety about your heart.

As you read on in (I hope) a relaxed and unhurried manner, you will feel some release of anxiety simply because you recognize yourself in some of the case histories of patients with fears similar to yours. You will learn what to expect from your doctor and also from yourself in this process of rehabilitation.

Dr. Campbell Moses, a medical director of the American Heart Association, once said, "I don't think there's a man over fifty-five who doesn't wonder if he has heart disease."

True. But I go a step further. There are no age boundaries. The anxious heart may beat in the young as well as in the elderly.

The main question for each reader to answer is this: Are your symptoms those of real heart disease or are they imaginary? Or both?

For many who read *Your Heart Is Stronger Than You Think,* the premise may turn into an accepted fact. Surely 15 to 20 million cardiophobes are not all beyond assistance. All I ask is your patience, an open mind, and willing cooperation. Peace of mind is an essential ingredient of peace of heart.

Meanwhile, here is how I propose to help:

In Part I, attention will be given to the various aspects of the ideal doctor–patient relationship. You will learn that you and your doctor are partners. To be successful, each individual must carry his fair share of responsibility. In addition, I will demonstrate the role of fear, anxiety, and "nerves" in creating symptoms that simulate the pain and discomfort of organic heart disease.

Part II will be devoted to practical information and specific advice about what to do for your "heart trouble." Do you think you have a heart cough? Are you certain that only a weak heart will produce palpitation and skips? Are you suspicious that the indigestion you had the other day was really "acute indigestion"—a heart attack? Is your fatigue really due to a weak heart or to something overlooked in your way of life (insufficient diet, oversmoking, overworking)? Is your shortness of breath actual difficulty in breathing or a form of hyperventilation that simulates heart disease? Do you have a murmur that worries you?

Scores of symptoms may have convinced you that you have heart "disease." My task will be to convince you that it may only be heart "trouble," and most often completely curable.

Part III treats of some special aspects of coronary disease, revealing the relationship of high and low blood pressure to heart problems, while also discussing rheumatic and congenital heart disease.

In Part IV readers will find more than two score practical pointers specifically aimed at making life more pleasant for those men and women who suffer from organic heart disease, and at helping them to avoid heart complications.

Peter J. Steincrohn, M.D., F.A.C.P.

Coral Gables, Florida
January, 1970

PART I

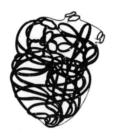

THE IDEAL
DOCTOR-PATIENT
RELATIONSHIP

1.

YOUR HEART AND
CHRONIC ANXIETY

Have you ever hated your doctor? There may have been good reason for it. Doctor–patient relationships are like parent–child relations. Love may suddenly turn into fleeting hate.

One harassed, dejected young housewife told me: "Sometimes I hate my doctor and sometimes I love him. Now, how can you account for that?"

I answered that I'd have a much better chance guessing it was the butler who committed the crime in a mystery tale: Not knowing her well nor her doctor, I could only answer with generalities that might not apply to her case.

As a doctor, I've been hated and loved—often by the same patients. I think it is easy to explain. We doctors are really father figures. And you know how children who love their fathers can also hate them at times—especially when they are having an unpleasant session with their fathers or being punished for some act of disobedience.

There are many reasons for loving one's doctor. He brings your husband or your wife through a dangerous attack of coronary thrombosis, or performs an emergency operation which saves your parent, or he delivers a sweet,

3

new addition to the family. How can you hate a man like that?

Well, you may turn on him months or years later because he doesn't come out in answer to a night call. Or you may think his bill is exorbitant. Or you may be annoyed because the magazines on his waiting-room table are several months old.

As in all relationships, love and hate are closely affiliated. One man hates his doctor because he says, "No more cigarettes," but the next patient loves him for it because "he takes such an interest in my welfare." One woman loves her doctor because he is the "quiet, understanding type," and another because he is the "talkative, outgoing physician." What pleases one patient will upset the next.

Almost as bad as parental punishment of the child is the calm assertion of the physician to the anxious patient: "There's nothing wrong with you." The patient often leaves the office like the spanked child—confused, frustrated and angry.

I recall a thirty-one-year-old magazine editor I saw early in my practice. He was dark-haired, slender but with good shoulders and a quick, impatient manner. He visited my office because he had become disenchanted with his former doctor. I asked him why.

"I was a perfectly healthy fellow until about three months ago," he told me. "I began to get heart skips that frightened me awfully. I thought I was going to die. They came every day and night. Soon they interfered with my work and sleep. I certainly wasn't imagining them. My doctor took all kinds of expensive tests. When he was through, guess what he said? 'There's nothing wrong with you. There's no need for you to come back!' Can you imagine a doctor turning a frightened patient loose without even

4

prescribing for him? What he seemed to be telling me was that I imagine the skips or exaggerate them. I used to like him. Frankly, I hate him now for saying, 'There's nothing wrong,' and letting me go."

In effect, that was his story. What could I, as a young doctor, hope to accomplish after an experienced clinician hadn't found the reason for his heart skips?

Fortunately, as an eager, beginning practitioner I had one thing in my favor—sufficient time to listen to him patiently. We sat together for at least an hour during that first visit. He talked about himself, his business problems, and his marital life. He admitted smoking close to three packs of cigarettes a day and drinking "more beer than he should" because he was tense and worried about risking most of his savings in a questionable business venture.

His physical examination was negative. His heart was strong. Before he left the office, and on his own decision, he resolved to sacrifice the few hundred dollars he had put up for an option. He called off the deal to save the wear and tear on his mind.

He phoned me a week later to say the skips had disappeared soon after he had stopped smoking and drinking. He thanked me "for listening" when he had been in my office. "I feel like a new man," he said.

I've often told associates, residents, and interns that, when a person "hurts" in one way or another, there's a reason—even if all physical and laboratory examinations are negative.

When a patient complains, there's always something wrong somewhere. Never tell him, "There's nothing wrong with you." Heart worry, for example, can be more exhausting than a broken leg.

Each one of us has his own private worry or fear. When people realize this they not only bear their own anxieties with more patience, but they have compassion for any of their acquaintances who have developed so-called "ridiculous fears."

Fear is as natural an impulse as hunger or thirst. Charles Berg, M.D., said, "There is constantly some degree of morbid anxiety in every normal life." (I tell people to cheer up. They have a lot of company.)

Edward Weiss, another M.D., wrote, "The anxiety neurosis, in its varying degrees, is probably the most frequent disorder of civilized life."

How and why does heart fear begin? Where does it originate? These are the questions that stricken people ask who suddenly (or perhaps gradually) lose touch with their former carefree ways of life.

I have often written that apparently "strong-minded" individuals should never laugh derisively at such scared "weaklings." For the problem is not a matter of strength or backbone or weakness of character. If life gets too rough or the strains grow too hard, not one of us can safely say we will never fall into chronic anxiety that focuses upon the heart—or elsewhere.

James Boswell quotes Aristotle as follows: "Why is it that all men who have excelled in philosophy, in politics, in poetry, or in the arts, have been subject to melancholy?" Then Boswell proceeds to disagree with him by stating, "Melancholy or hypochondria, like the fever or gout, or any other disease, is incident to all sorts of men, from the wisest to the most foolish."

For example, here is a housewife in her middle thirties with two lovely preschool children and an above-average husband. She says in a letter recently sent to me:

> For the past month I've become very nervous about taking any trips outside of my home such as shopping, dining out, making visits to recreational areas like

plays, musicals, movies, because I'm concerned about my heart. I get weak and faint and my heart palpitates. I think I'm going to die. When some event is planned I worry so about participating that the children suffer. I can't enjoy playing or listening to them. My husband's position requires moves every few years and I've become anxious about uprooting the family so often. His position also requires a great deal of socializing, but I am concerned about these obligations, and can't seem to cope with them.

What guidance can one give such a hapless individual? One can't prescribe specific treatment by mail. There is no one supertranquilizer or other medication that will remove her fears as if erasing a blackboard. The best solution is for her to find a doctor who will help her fight this anxiety about her heart.

Anxiety states sometimes begin with an acute attack of fear. It is called an anxiety attack. The person feels "something awful is going to happen." He is assailed by sudden shortness of breath, palpitations, weakness, sweating, nausea, and dizziness.

It is natural for the individual to conclude that some serious heart disability is the reason, rather than attribute the symptoms to an emotional difficulty. Sometimes, in addition to palpitation, there is pain in the left side of the chest, and a runaway heart. Such an attack is usually followed by nervousness, irritability, ringing in the ears, insomnia, sighing respiration, and chronic fatigue.

In some patients this anxiety state about the heart begins gradually. It often affects those who are apparently happy and who haven't a worry in the world. It's the doctor's job to discover the underlying reason for these heart fears.

Treatment varies. It consists of psychotherapy, encouragement, tranquilizers, and energizers; and repeated defenses built by patient and doctor against surrender. As I said, the fight is often prolonged, but defeat is not inevitable.

In some people, chronic anxiety about the heart lasts only for a few weeks; in others the frightening symptoms linger for months and years.

The main thing is to have faith that you will ultimately overcome the anxiety, however discouraged you feel now. Doctors can help just so much. Success or failure depends, in most instances, upon the patient's willingness to get off the floor time and again and keep punching. Sometimes, prayer is the only solution.

When will the self-appointed brave people of this world develop an understanding and sympathy for their more fearful brethren? It is especially difficult for the scared ones when members of their own family treat them with contempt and ridicule.

For example, here is a confession by a forty-two-year-old housewife:

> I have a problem concerning water and very high bridges over water. I am very much afraid of them and I will not cross over on them. I've felt this way as long as I can remember. When I get close to a bridge, I shiver all over and suffer the most frightful heart palpitations. When I look out at the vast body of water with nothing around it like trees, shrubs or other things, I feel as if I'm going to be swallowed up by it or suffer a heart attack. My husband accuses me of ruining his life because of what he calls my "silly fears."

I told her that her husband should consider himself fortunate in not having some kind of phobia—big or little. He should know that her fears are real and not "silly."

8

I also advised her to ask her doctor to suggest some psychiatrist in her area to whom she might go for treatment and I passed along the name of one particular psychiatrist whom I know quite well.

This unfortunate woman had a mixture of phobias and apprehension. For instance, she suffered from agorophobia (fear of open space), ochophobia (fear of automobiles), kinesophobia (fear of vehicles), thalassophobia (fear of the sea), and gephyrophobia (crossing bridges).

In a situation of this nature the family physician should recognize his limitations and the need for additional help in solving the patient's problems. The many phobias plaguing this woman were sufficient evidence that her anxiety was not easily explainable or treated. Her surge of frightening tensions deserved expert care.

Subsequently she was referred to the psychiatrist I had suggested. He, in turn, later reported to me that she had recently taken some auto rides that involved crossing high bridges, without experiencing fearsome anxiety reactions.

"How did you accomplish it?" I asked.

"It's a long story," he replied. "It begins with an unfortunate psychosexual experience that touched off the anxiety. Now that she is beginning to understand her problem, she feels better."

Periodically I write about common fears so that the "emotionally strong" will realize that family members or friends who complain are not just making up these obsessions to get sympathy. They are as real as can be, and scientists have attached various erudite tags (some are real tongue-twisters) to each peculiar anxiety feeling. However, one fear leads them all: *cardiophobia* (fear of one's heart capacity).

As Dr. Weiss has said, "In spite of the enormous incidence of cardiovascular disease, the majority of patients

9

who have symptoms referred to the heart region do not have evidence of organic heart disease."

The reason is not hard to find. From time immemorial the heart has been the traditional seat of emotions, and hence acts as a focal point for anxiety. Our language is rich with expressions linking the heart with courage or the lack of it, with love, and with hate.

But patients with distressing symptoms often say, "It must be my heart. I'm not nervous. Yet, I have this palpitation and heart weakness. If it's not my nerves, then there must be something physically wrong."

Long ago, Freud emphasized that attacks of palpitation, heart irregularity, rapid heart action—due to vasomotor instability or autonomic imbalance (nervous disturbances) —are not always accompanied by recognizable anxiety.

The patient doesn't always realize he is nervous and anxious. This is one reason why he so often regards his symptoms as undisputed indications of physical disease of the heart. He can't imagine that emotions alone would cause all his apprehensions. The anxiety attached to his heart's behavior is often totally unknown to the patient who is certain he has heart disease, until the doctor convinces him his problem is in his mind. Mind? What is it?

In brief, here is the anatomy of the mind:

You have a conscious and an unconscious mind. In the conscious is the greater part of your ego; and in your unconscious is the id. Between your ego and your id stands the superego. As your ego and id are forever sparring, it is the superego's job to act as arbiter.

Your id is the caveman principle in all human beings. It is a vast, uncharted region of powerful unconscious urges, instincts, and desires. It is uninhibited. All it wants to do is have fun. It detests such shackles as laws of behavior.

But your ego is your region of perceptivity. It is your immediate contact with reality and with your environment.

Whenever your id tries to break loose in some intemperate, impulsive pleasure it is the job of your superego to hold it in check. And what a job it has! For the id is not concerned with what you think of people or what people think of you. It is untamed in manner and is a creature of lusts. It wants what it wants when it wants it. And its demands create a daily battle because your ego and superego find that their own energy flows out of this id which they are forever trying to keep within "civilized bounds."

If the tests of strength between these various forces buried deep inside you are not too unbearable, they are easily resolved. However, if the conscious and the unconscious are locked in daily battles of some magnitude, the result is conflict. And this eight-letter word forms the basis of what we call psychoneurosis.

One of several definitions of psychoneurosis, and an excellent one, is that given by Dr. Samuel B. Hadden: "To me a psychoneurosis is a group of symptoms which may be physical, mental, or both, which develops in an individual when he is incapable of dealing successfully with the circumstances in his life at a given time. His powers of adaptability are inadequate in the face of the complexities of the present situation."

It is because we have come to realize more and more (although Hippocrates knew it thousands of years ago) that the mind and the body are interdependent that we attach so much importance to "psychosomatics." It may be a new term, but it is an old, established medical idea. It does not mean that we should study the soma (body) less, but the psyche (mind) more.

Many disbelievers are still around. They say, "Don't you

11

think that doctors have gone overboard in their belief that emotions have so much to do with health?"

Personally, I don't think we have gone overboard often enough in our management of disease. Otherwise, we would put more effort in straightening out a patient's emotions rather than in just giving him pills and diets. How can I convince you disbelievers? Let's consider some simple facts:

Have you ever had to go to the bathroom often before a school examination? (Emotions are acting on bowel or bladder.)

Have you ever slipped and "almost" toppled over a high cliff? Sudden fear dilated your pupils, raced your heart, made you break into a sweat. (Emotions are acting on eyes, heart, and skin.)

Have you ever paced up and down a corridor before going in to see a particular individual about some important matter such as getting a job or putting over a big business deal? Did the palms of your hands sweat? Was your mouth dry? (Emotions are acting on your hands and mouth.)

Do you recall how your stomach bunched up after an argument so that you couldn't sit down to eat? (Emotions are acting on your gastric juices and the muscles of your stomach.)

Have you ever said, "He gives me a headache." (Emotions!)

I have been supplying examples of the physiological and anatomical changes that take place momentarily when emotions run berserk. Believe me, then, when I say that intense emotion—either sudden or protracted—can produce changes in the physical being and cause symptoms of heart trouble (heart phobias, palpitation, pain, shortness of breath, among others) that is imaginary and not due to actual heart disease. Of course such emotions can also induce reactions that result in high blood pressure, coronary disease, ulcer, hyperthyroidism, ulcerative colitis, and many other serious medical conditions.

It is for these reasons that the competent doctor is not the one who treats the disease but the one who treats the "whole man." He must evaluate your emotional as well as your physical health. Here is a letter I received about a year ago from a frightened and despondent young woman:

> Dear Dr. Steincrohn:
>
> I am solely interested in easing my mind. I am twenty, married and go to work. I have been running to doctors for almost six years now with little success. In each case the diagnosis is the same—nerves! But I keep on feeling bad and it is now getting to the point where I cannot bear living like this. Always fighting to catch my breath. Worrying about a weak heart.
>
> I cannot understand how nerves alone can make a person feel the way I do constantly. Maybe you have come across others with this same problem. My symptoms most surely indicate some serious heart disease. I am forever groggy and dizzy. I am extremely despondent and have the urge to scream or run to get away from myself. I break out in cold sweats. My legs go weak and once went completely numb for a few days. My throat feels tight. My muscles ache as if I'm coming down with influenza at times.
>
> But what frightened me most is waking up at night with palpitations and the fear that my heart will stop beating. I have had three electrocardiograms and two heart X rays, but they showed nothing wrong.
>
> Can a doctor tell if there's something seriously wrong

with the heart if the patient is just "neurotic?" I feel as if I am alone in my problem and that nobody can help me. Can you give me some comfort and advice, please?

As for giving some comfort, what could I say other than that I have seen thousands of patients with symptoms similar to hers? After careful examinations I, too, found her free of organic heart disease. And, as she put it, "nerves" was the underlying cause of the discomforts she and these thousands of other patients suffered.

However, I told Eleanore F. that the important point for us all to remember is that we must try to rule out every type of real heart disease before pinning the diagnostic tag of imaginary heart trouble on any patient. I had seen a number of patients who had been treated as psychoneurotics for years ("just plain nerves") but who, on careful examination and study, later proved to be suffering from undulant fever, an overactive thyroid, or from some other organic disease. Excerpts from the rest of my answering letter follow.

I think your mistake is in flitting from doctor to doctor. There doesn't seem to be one whom you can call your friend as well as doctor. You should choose one who is patient and of good scientific ability (you can get a doctor's qualifications from the secretary of your local medical society or from local hospitals). The efficient doctor will first study you completely to rule out organic heart disease. Not until then may he arrive at the provisional diagnosis of psychoneurosis—and prescribe proper treatment.

If your trouble is purely "nerves," be thankful you do not have a life-shortening ailment. It is true that a neurosis can be stubborn and resist treatment for months (and years), but have faith that you will at

last overcome it and improve—as so many similar patients have in the past.

Not until many weeks later did this patient admit that
her husband was a weekend alcoholic who mistreated her
and the children. Since she had kept this facet of her life
locked within her, the tensions manifested themselves as
heart symptoms. Her improvement finally came after her
husband joined Alcoholics Anonymous and gave up drinking.

Many recover, although the ever-present belief in the
mind of the patient with chronic anxiety about his heart
is that he will never improve: "How is it ever possible to
feel well again? How can anyone with such fears as mine
ever hope to live like a normal human being again?" Such
are the questions the patient asks his doctor and continu-
ally asks himself.

In spite of this common denominator of hopelessness,
I keep telling patients that there is, indeed hope. I admit
that in many cases it is a long process that taxes their
willpower and moral strength; but the determination to
overcome anxieties and fears nevertheless can triumph.

Chronic anxiety about the heart is not a hopeless condition. I receive many letters from such sufferers and have
personally treated thousands of patients whose universal
complaint was that they were doomed to go on living as
invalids. However, the condition can be overcome if you
have the will to fight it and the persistence to find a sympathetic doctor to lean on when things seem almost unbearable. Consider this letter I recently received from one
of my readers:

> You wrote in your column that chronic anxiety about
> one's heart can be one of "mankind's greatest trials."
> You are so right. For months there was never a morn-

15

ing that I was not surprised (and relieved) to find that I was still alive—that my heart had not given out while I was asleep.

I want to send my best wishes, hope, and encouragement to a Mrs. X. who wrote to you about her sufferings. I've been through the same misery, I had the added burden of deep depression. Yet, I am happy to report that I have made a complete recovery. Life has become not only more endurable, but enjoyable.

Go on talking freely to your doctor. Take whatever treatment and medication he prescribes. Have faith in God and in your doctor. I, too, was discouraged, because progress is so slow. But it can be made. Slowly you will come to rely more on your heart's basic strength. I hope you will soon be well, and that life will be a joy for you again.

Too many self-styled heroes around take considerable gambles with their lives. They are fatalists who look down on people who maintain a careful watch on their health. They say, "Oh, you're always running to a doctor for every little ache or pain."

Many hypochondriacs make unnecessary trips to the doctor's office because of abnormal anxieties. However, there are probably just as many persons who are scared about their hearts, but are afraid to acknowledge their fear to others.

The greatest difference between a hypochondriac and the rest of us is that the hypochondriac is scared and admits it.

For example, I have treated many patients with angina who told me they didn't come for advice until after they had had symptoms of chest pain on exertion for many months. When I asked them why they had not consulted me earlier, the customary reply was, "I guess I wanted to be a hero and suffer in silence. The truth is I was scared but afraid to admit it."

I repeated what I have told many others: It is better to be a live hypochondriac at eighty than a dead hero at forty. Accordingly, if you are abnormally heart-conscious (which is a refined way of saying you're scared of your heart), visit your doctor immediately and let him determine the actual condition of that most important organ in your body. The chances are more than likely that he'll find it normal, and that you have been one of the vast multitude of men and women who have imaginary heart trouble or are running heart-scared.

On the other hand, if he discovers some heart impairment, he can prescribe medication and give you specific advice about how to cope with the condition with a minimum of discomfort and alteration of your regular living routine.

Whenever I am frustrated in establishing an effective treatment for a patient, I never hesitate to consider a suggestion from another sufferer. The science of medicine should never hold the art of medicine in contempt. It is for this reason that I occasionally reprint letters from patients who have been helped and hope to help others. The following missive is particularly revealing:

> I was a prisoner in a "neurotic hell" for twenty-nine seemingly interminable years. The several doctors I had within the period tried everything. Here is a very incomplete list: long fasts, many varied diets, periods of sexual abstinence, innumerable enemas, anterior pituitary injections for several months, two different psychiatric clinics for months, all kinds of vitamins, iron injections, rest and more rest, sunbaths, long walks, the milk diet, three or four kinds of sleeping pills, various tranquilizers. You name it and chances

17

are I have tried it! I even tried autosuggestion, with only temporary benefit. Yet, I continued to worry about my heart.

Finally, six months ago, in desperation, I resolved to try autosuggestion once more but with more persistence than I had used before. I had often thought that if I could become truly religious it might be the answer. But I just didn't know how.

I am now convinced that the major cause of anxiety neurosis is negative thinking. One can get so used to it that he is hardly aware he's doing it. In a way it is analagous to the narcotic habit and may not be greatly easier to break. But it must be done if one hopes to be well and happy. Positive thinking finally gets easier after a few weeks of hard application.

It is my opinion that autosuggestion is fine but, to be fully effective, it must be positive thinking slanted in a religious direction. In fact, positive thinking gave me the first real entree to religion.

There are many fine books on positive thinking, if one looks for them. The best one I know, for my own use, is *Let Go and Let God* by Albert E. Cliffe. I have underlined many of its positive statements in ink and I read them over and over again. His book actually states that the way to develop faith is by positive thinking and I know he is right.

Also, Dr. Norman Vincent Peale is a well-known advocate of positive thinking. He published a booklet called *Thought Conditioners* several years ago. I use it several times a day and wouldn't be without it.

I have known a good many people who endured what was known as cardiac neurosis. And, believe me, I know how they suffered. But they, like I, have found the answer I have been giving you. Life has just begun again for all of us. (Incidentally, positive thinking leading to faith in God is wonderful for "normal" people, too.)

2.

THYROID PROBLEMS AND
LOW BLOOD SUGAR

My experience has been that two of the most commonly overlooked diagnoses causing anxiety are thyroid trouble (mostly the underactive variety) and abnormally low blood sugar (called hypoglycemia).

If you have been labeled a cardiac neurotic and told that "only nerves" are the reasons for your complaints, then you have the right to ask for a consultation. Especially if your doctor has not taken tests to determine your thyroid function and has not suggested blood-sugar tolerance tests to rule out abnormally low blood sugar (often called idiopathic hypoglycemia).

Causes of hypoglycemia vary. In some few patients the cause is easily determined as being a tumor in the pancreas (an islet tumor) which secretes too much insulin and causes the low blood sugar. An operation usually relieves such patients.

However, the most commonly overlooked type is idiopathic hypoglycemia (cause unknown). What is most important is finding the typically "flat" blood-sugar curves during the blood-sugar tolerance examination—taking

19

blood tests every hour for five hours after drinking a measured amount of sweets.

Such symptoms as faintness and palpitation—which suggest the possibility of heart impairment to many people —disappear in many patients after they stop smoking. There have been other reports that alcohol produces hypoglycemia in sensitive patients; in others, coffee seems to lower the blood sugar.

Dr. Martin S. Buehler, of Dallas, Texas, in a paper in the journal *Lancet* says:

> Certainly, by the number of cases that I have been able to collect over a relatively short period, this condition [hypoglycemia] must be extremely common; it is very important as well, inasmuch as most of these cases are misdiagnosed, often as neuroses, and many patients have even been referred for psychiatric therapy. All of this seems quite tragic to me, since the vast majority of them can be rapidly cured of their symptoms or completely kept under control by correct therapy.

The basis of treatment for hypoglycemia, it is generally agreed, must be a decrease in the intake of carbohydrates and an increase in proteins. Some patients may need sedatives and large amounts of vitamins, especially of nicotinic acid, and adrenal cortical extract.

"You're a neurotic!" Thousands of Americans are wearing that tag. Basically well adjusted and not suffering from any deep-seated neurosis, they still complain.

For example, take the case of a forty-two-year-old electrical engineer who was formerly tough-minded enough to meet any emergency. During the past few months he has become a "complainer"—a "neurotic." He's always running scared.

He has told family and friends that he is plagued by weak spells during the day. He suddenly gets "awfully hungry and faint." He says he sweats a lot and sometimes actually finds himself trembling for no reason. He is afraid that he will collapse of heart failure wherever he is—at home, on the street, or behind the wheel of his car. He has discovered that the only thing that brings temporary relief is taking a few chocolate candies.

At last he is prodded into seeing his doctor who is a good diagnostician. Because of our man's sudden hunger and spells of faintness and sweating, the doctor suspects hyperinsulinism with low blood sugar. The patient returns for special blood-sugar tolerance tests. The blood-sugar levels are abnormally low and confirm the doctor's suspicions.

Further investigation indicates the presence of an "islet" tumor in the pancreas. The patient comes to surgery, the tumor is removed and the so-called "neurotic" is normal again. And all the apparent symptoms of heart disease miraculously go away. Here then was another of the millions of individuals with imaginary heart disease.

Unfortunately, all cases of hypoglycemia do not have so happy an ending. Many go undiscovered because they are simply overlooked. Others, who experience discomfort after a period of fasting (during the night), discover their most revealing symptoms at breakfast time. The nervousness, weakness, and sweating disappear right after breakfast. They have more spells during the day as the blood sugar falls. However, once the diagnosis is made, a special high-protein diet improves the condition.

Here is the interesting case history of an office manager with heart anxiety, which indicates how symptoms may vary when blood sugar is abnormally low:

For months, this man had been treated as a hopeless

21

hypochondriac. After a while, he dreaded going to the doctor and being patted on the back patronizingly, while being told his problem was his nerves, not his heart. After a while he felt guilty about complaining to his wife and children because they began to regard him as a lazy lout who was trying to shirk his responsibilitity to support his family.

Finally, he visited a young doctor who said he had a hunch. Although physical examination showed nothing special, he had a notion that laboratory tests might clear up the mystery.

He ordered a blood-sugar tolerance test which revealed that the patient suffered from low blood sugar (hypoglycemia). In addition to that, he had a condition called narcolepsy, which was the reason why the office manager had been so sleepy and tired all the time.

He was put on a low carbohydrate-high protein diet and was given pills that dispelled the heart palpitations and the sleepy feelings. Within a few weeks he became an entirely different person.

Narcolepsy alone is bad enough. Add the discomforts of hypoglycemia, and it all adds up to the unhappy person just described.

I have seen fat, sleepy people who were called hypochondriacs by family and business associates, yet were innocent sufferers. They really were always exhausted. It wasn't their imagination. They had true anxiety, depression, "heart weakness," headaches, insomnia, nervousness, tremor of the fingers. But they did *not* have organic heart disease.

All the symptoms were due to abnormally low blood sugar. High-protein diet helped straighten them out. As for the sleepy people plagued by narcolepsy, they were fully alert within days after taking special drugs (i.e.,

Benzedrine, Dexedrine, Ritalin, etc.) that sparked life into their drooping eyelids.

If you have been labeled a neurotic, I think the designation is unfair unless you have been given the full benefit of blood-sugar studies by a competent laboratory. As for stubborn, continued drowsiness, this deserves the consideration that narcolepsy might be present.

Often doctors don't get a chance to really help a patient when the latter does come for a consultation because of the fear of being ridiculed for relating what may seem to be silly symptoms. It is for this reason that I urge patients and readers not to withhold any information from their doctors. By the same token, the medical practitioner should not disparage patients who seek help or ask questions which may have no sound basis in medical fact.

What I have been saying deserves further emphasis, for it is all too common for patients to keep quiet when they should be unburdening themselves. In being so taciturn (because they are "afraid to talk") they make it difficult for themselves and their physician, and it is important to remember that no one is immune to the onset of anxiety about the heart or other organs. The blow can strike suddenly and unexpectedly.

Quite some time ago I wrote in one of my newspaper columns, "If man could see tomorrow's newspaper today, he would turn first to the stock quotations, and forget about looking on the obituary page."

I asked myself what I meant when I said that. What it does, I believe, is draw a distinction between the importance of riches and actual survival. I am not at all surprised that man takes his health and life for granted while he, like King Midas, lives only to increase his stock of gold.

23

For years I've been trying to tell people that nothing is more important than health and life itself; that riches, for riches' sake, are of secondary importance.

An editor friend of mine, Leonard M. Leonard, once wrote: "Think how happy you'd be if you lost everything you have right now and then got it back again."

Well, you may get all your material possessions back if you are lucky, but it doesn't usually work that way with health. Illness, emotional or physical (or both), leaves its scars. And preventive medicine can do much to spare you from illness.

Whether or not you waste your heart's strength may depend upon your philosophy of life. If you are a fatalist you may overwork, overeat, oversmoke, overdrink, overplay, overworry—and underrelax. You may wring so much emotion out of your body that you wear it down to a palpitating frazzle. Instead of pacing your heart for the long journey, you spring from day to day. The result is physical or emotional exhaustion.

In either case, whether you develop real heart disease or imaginary heart trouble, you will need professional help to guide you back to a way of life that is satisfactory and fulfilled. You can't do it alone, You will need a good doctor.

Sometimes the question of imaginary heart trouble stands in the way of marriage as much as does real heart disease. I recall one young college senior who came to me with the following story. Unsmiling and apparently under emotional control she tried to hide what was indeed a problem to her. She was an attractive blonde, long-legged, full-bosomed with finely molded features. Her manner appeared almost hostile as she began speaking:

"My boy friend, who is twenty-nine, had a nervous breakdown seven years ago while in college. I have just

24

learned he is still under a doctor's care and sees him regularly. According to his family, he keeps worrying that he has heart disease even though his doctor assures him he has a normal heart.

"We are planning to get married and I am wondering if this is serious or not. We are not formally engaged and I haven't been able to bring myself to ask him to tell me some of the details and answers to my doubts. I feel I might be prying into something of a personal nature which might be a sore spot with him.

"Could you tell me if it is possible he has not fully recovered from his breakdown? We have been dating steadily for the past six months and he seems normal except he occasionally says that his heart is getting lazy. What would you do?"

I told her what I have advised many in similar circumstances: "I have made it a point never to tell someone, 'Do get married' or 'Don't get married,' for medical reasons. For example, the term nervous breakdown might signify anything from overfatigue due to stress (and temporary neurosis) to actual serious psychosis like schizophrenia or manic disease.

"The ones involved should make the decisions themselves. However, they should be given all the facts before they decide. In your case I might be doing both you and your young man a disservice by saying 'no.' He may never be bothered again by the breakdown he suffered years ago.

"On the other hand, by not warning you to be careful before you make your decision I might indirectly be the cause of giving you a lifetime of unhappiness. Because it is possible, you know, that he has much more than imaginary heart trouble. It is possible that he has a serious mental disorder. But I don't know.

"Have your own doctor examine him and give you the

facts. Marriage and happiness, being the gambles they are, should not be forced unknowingly to carry the added burden of serious illness in one or both partners. Each should go into it with eyes open."

In the next chapter I propose to indicate the minimum support you can expect from a competent physician. Later I will provide specific advice on how to live with a heart that may be stronger than you think. Nevertheless, as a patient, you also have a job to do:

If you are "heart-scared," do something about it now. Your need is not to *wonder* but to *know*. Make an appointment with an able physician; he will help you combat your chronic anxiety.

Here is the crux of it all. Having been told your heart is normal, after a thorough evaluation, try to discard whatever fears you may have when your doctor hands down a verdict of "heart not guilty."

Accept it with relief. Believe him. Otherwise, you will soon be on the crowded medical merry-go-round, feeling worse and worse as you try doctor after doctor—always disbelieving that your heart is normal. (Ultimately, such thinking may be the green arrow to the psychiatrist's couch.)

3.

YOUR DOCTOR MUST HELP

Doctors should not disparage good bedside manners—especially when they are treating a patient who lives in fear that his heart may fail at any time in the near future. Such people die the proverbial thousand deaths. Every day is a joust with the forces of extermination, though their hearts may be normal.

Although this is a century when scientific medicine is making tremendous headway in diagnosis and treatment of cardiac ailments, I remind my colleagues that good old-fashioned heart is still as important as head in the management of heart patients (imaginary or real). Robot and computer medicine is here to stay, but it should be subservient to the doctor and not lead him by the nose.

You can't be a good doctor unless you feel for the patient. Empathy is the ubiquitous name for it. I keep emphasizing the importance of this to younger practitioners who sometimes are more interested in evaluating computer results or eagerly reading a laboratory sheet than taking the patient's pulse or asking him, "Did you sleep well last night? Do you have any pain?"

Bedside manner isn't something that you study, it's

something that you are. The patient soon sees through artificial sympathy or feigned interest; he detects it when the doctor's thoughts wander.

What is a good bedside manner? It is a combination of qualities—inherent in the doctor's personality or learned because of intense interest in his patients.

The good doctor must have tact. He must know how to handle the patient and his family firmly, yet gently. He must be cheerful. He must inspire faith in the patient's future. He must radiate confidence, which comes of an inner dependence upon his own knowledge and ability.

The good doctor must be patient and unhurried. He must have large ears, to listen long and hard to the patient's detailed and sometimes rambling explanation of his discomforts and overburdening anxieties. When the patient leaves your office or when you walk away from his bedside, the patient should feel that he has a friend as well as a professional adviser. Such a doctor—and there are many, in spite of the medical profession's jaded image —is a godsend to the sick. Especially to the frightened cardiophobe who wonders whether he will last the day.

One common complaint of patients goes like this: "I like my doctor except for one thing. He doesn't give me any time. When I leave, I don't feel that I've had my money's worth."

I don't deny that the fault is often the doctor's. Whatever the reason—lateness for a hospital appointment and a full outer office, the need for making an emergency call, apparent disinterest—I agree that the patient has a right to feel slighted. But there are times when the patient himself is responsible for not getting everything he should out of his office visit.

For example, suppose you arrive for an appointment, and the doctor is relaxed, unhurried, and intent on obtaining a good history of your illness. But getting you to talk is almost like having to pull teeth. Either for reasons of prudery or actual loss of memory, because you become so nervous in a doctor's office, you fail to give him the necessary leads or clues in tracking down real or imaginary heart trouble.

It was Dr. Joseph F. Montague who originated the phrase which is now a common part of the language: "You do not get ulcers from what you eat. You get ulcers from what is eating you."

In their book *Psychosomatic Medicine,* Dr. Weiss and Dr. English explain the rebellious acts of our various body organs. They say that patients who cannot find a normal outlet for their emotions, by word or act, will inevitably produce tensions in the heart, stomach, intestines, etc., by which these organs will talk a kind of "organ language."

For example, the stomach will get upset and be saying: "I can't stomach this." Intestines will become loose and be saying, "I've got to get rid of this." The heart will skip and jump and ache as if to say, "Oh, for the days when I was strong and healthy."

Weiss and English continue with the following observations:

> The more we can persuade our patients to talk about themselves as human beings rather than as medical cases, the sooner we will come to understand their symptoms of emotional origin. . . . Medicine had its real beginning in the study of man at the dissecting table. Let us continue with the study of man not only as an anatomical and physiological mechanism but as a human being possessed of loves and hates, urges and passions, capable of disturbing his soul and his body.

I recall a young secretary who came to see me at least

29

a half dozen times for "headaches." She was a pretty, frail-looking girl, her fine features marred by a sense of strain that also shadowed her eyes. It seemed to require a conscious effort for her to smile, Finally, after an interval of several weeks, she paid me another visit.

"How is the headache problem lately?"

She frowned and said, "I guess I may as well own up to it, doctor. What I've really come for is to be reassured about my heart. This has been my main worry.

"I haven't told you because you'd think it silly for me to worry simply because I nursed my mother with a heart condition for months before she died. I think my symptoms are just like hers, but I have been afraid to get the true verdict."

In this young woman's case dramatic improvement followed a complete cardiac evaluation that indicated her heart was normal.

"The reason I believe in my heart now," she later informed me, "is because I've had electrocardiograms, X rays and all the rest. All that my previous examinations consisted of were hasty layings-on of the stethoscope. I had no confidence in the findings."

Incidentally, her headaches vanished when her nervous tension about her heart abated.

I also remember the case of a middle-aged but very active attorney who was anxious about having coronary disease because his father and uncle had died from it several years before. He confessed to me that he had withheld his fears for many months because he thought he would be ridiculed if he even mentioned them to a doctor.

The vague chest pains of which he complained and his fear of heart disease evaporated within minutes after a heart tracing was taken indicating that his heart was normal.

30

When I had completed the examination, he smiled with relief and shook my hand. "That's all I've been waiting to learn," he said. "You can't imagine how frightened I've been having to face up to the verdict."

An architect was certain that his nervousness about his heart would lead to something much worse. It was months before he admitted that a grandparent was in a mental institution following a coronary attack. He confessed that he had been ashamed to let me peek into the skeleton closet. His nervousness and heart symptoms had disappeared by the time he left the office after I convinced him that this grandfather's illness was not hereditary.

Assuming that your doctor affords you all the time you need, be sure to take advantage of it. Do not allow nervousness to interfere with the necessary questions or the important revelations in your own and your family's history. It's your health. It's your life. You are paying for the doctor's time and experience. You have the right to ask questions and the obligation to reply with proper answers to his own questions.

When patients feel miserable, a good doctor encourages them to "get it out of their system." As I said, the name for it is "ventilate." Instead of talking it out with their doctor, minister, or friend, many persons stand in a corner somewhere and speak aloud their tribulations. There is also another way, which is effective for some people. For example, consider this letter I received from a woman in northern Minnesota:

> While lying here in my hospital bed, I find that by writing down my feelings and expressing my emotional upheaval, I begin to feel better and get back on an even keel. It may seem ridiculous, but it's true in my case. This is one of those forty-five-year-old's days when nobody loves me and everybody oppresses me and ab-

31

solutely no one understands me. I have real pains on my left side over my heart and nobody cares. I know I'm miserable and foolish but I can't help it. In fact, "I" is my whole world today. I have a crawly feeling up and down my spine. One minute I think I'll live, and the next I'm sure my heart will suddenly give out.

I look around me but I can't see the lady who has had a bad fracture of her leg and is in severe pain because it isn't healing properly. I can't see the man who faces a serious operation tomorrow. I can't see the young girl who has just lost her baby. Nor do I see the heartbroken woman whose husband died yesterday.

When I say, "I don't see them," I mean I'm too taken up with my own feelings. I will feel sympathy tomorrow. But today! That is dedicated to all my own problems. I grovel in the pit of despair because I can't do a single, solitary thing to stop this awful depression. But hold on! Believe it or not, now that I've written all this down I'm beginning to feel better. I think I'll dry my eyes and go over to talk to the young mother. Or maybe say a few words to the woman who is still too shocked to realize what it feels like to be a widow. For a few hours, at least, I'll thumb my nose at my heart.

There are other ways "of writing it down." So many patients complain that they do not get everything they should out of a visit to the doctor because they forget to ask pertinent questions. I tell such people there is a simple solution: Write down your questions before you arrive at his office and carry pad and pen to the doctor's office. Also write down his suggestions after he has examined you.

In that way you leave little room for misunderstanding.

Millions of dollars' worth of good advice is lost every year in doctors' offices simply because patients forget what the doctor said. I hope the following letter will give you the needed incentive to subscribe to the pen-and-pad habit:

> Some of us have a difficulty in telling facts when the subject is "me." It is probably a form of self-consciousness but it does exist.
>
> Our family doctor is also a close friend. And I have many reasons to think that technically and professionally he is all one could wish for in a doctor. Yet, on many occasions I have forgotten to tell him about some important matter. And almost invariably, I forget to ask for a prescription renewal. Yet, I have the reputation of having an exceptional memory.
>
> Neither has it been a case of office rush. (Heaven knows he spends too much time on my visits.) His office is always orderly and neat and in good taste, and his nurses have been extremely friendly and I have never had to worry about bills. Under such circumstances there's no reason why I shouldn't remember to tell and ask everything that is on my mind about my heart.
>
> I used to wonder why I was always forgetting things in the presence of doctors, but not anywhere else. It must be that most of us dislike talking about our intimate selves. In time it becomes so ingrained in our nature that we consciously preclude personal references.
>
> Many other patients must be like me in this manner. At last I solved the problem myself, by making advance notes of heart complaints I wanted to point out, then checking them off as we discussed them. And by taking notes of what my doctor said to me. Surely, I would still be a forgetful clam had I not adopted this method.

Patients are often concerned because they do not believe that their doctor is telling them the truth about their heart. Others complain that their doctor is a worrymonger. "When he explains your condition he worries you to death. Why aren't doctors more tactful?"

Sometimes we doctors are damned if we do and damned if we don't. The doctor–patient relationship is a fragile thing. Of course, much depends upon the innate tactfulness of your doctor. But you should remember that much depends upon you, too.

Like many medical practitioners, I have tried to be careful in explaining a patient's heart status, the outlook, and the treatment. But hard as you try, sometimes the patient is so inherently anxious about himself that anything you say may be magnified and distorted into something you didn't say at all. Often patients unconsciously close their ears to what they do not want to hear.

I recall one woman whose husband had serious heart disease. He was told how to live, what to do, and what not to do, and his wife knew, also, that he had an extremely serious form of angina pectoris.

At least, I thought she knew. When he died unexpectedly, her first words were: "Doctor, why didn't you tell me? Why didn't you warn me Jim was so sick?"

Not until months later did she visit me to say that she knew all along how ill he was, but just couldn't get herself to admit it. Here was the typical case of a doctor telling the truth, not keeping the patient guessing nor scaring the family to death. Yet the patient's family could not consciously accept the poor prognosis.

Most patients will be happier if they believe that the doctor is leveling with them instead of sugar-coating the diagnosis, the treatment, or the prognosis.

With few exceptions, I prefer to take the patient into my confidence. It's his health and his life, and he deserves to know. It is not fair to pussyfoot with him. I prefer to be called a worrymonger and have the patient know and follow directions and have a better chance to recover, than keep him ignorant of his condition so that he lives in false security.

If a patient comes to his doctor thinking he is well and has a physical examination, he should know if he has hidden illness. You may scare him half to death if you tell him you have discovered diabetes, but he'd better know. You may alarm him by suggesting a series of electrocardiograms to discover if his symptoms preclude organic heart disease, but he'd better know that, too.

If I had to choose between a doctor whom I disbelieved and one who was frank and friendly, I'd choose the latter. Once a patient loses faith in a doctor's integrity (in today's phrase—there is a credibility gap) he might as well go looking for another. Many patients would have been better off if their doctors had scared them into taking better care of themselves.

One day I was asked this question by an apprehensive patient who had consulted at least a dozen doctors, seeking relief and support she could not find. She was certain that she had heart disease, yet all the doctors agreed that she had a normal heart. She asked me: "Doctors get sick. Suppose you or someone in your family became very ill —or even thought they were ill—what kind of doctor would you like to have?" 1536939

First, I would like my doctor to be a fine human being with all that connotes. (Assuming, of course, that he had all the necessary scientific qualifications to be a competent practitioner.)

Is he compassionate? Do you get the feeling when you talk to him that here's a fellow who is truly sorry for you and one you can depend on to do everything possible to get you out of your mess?

35

Does he really listen? Or do you sense as you talk about your own complaints that his mind is on other matters— his golf game, the stock market, his own family problems. I'd like my doctor to have large ears that really listen.

Is he too confident and opinionated? I do not like or trust persons who talk and act as if they are God's gift to humanity—who are so sure of everything they do and say that they put up their backs at the very mention of consultation to get another medical opinion. I would like my doctor to be big enough to say that another doctor's viewpoint might be well worth having.

Is he conscientious? If he is, you will not have to wonder about his conduct of practice. You will know that he makes necessary house calls and night calls (or sees to it that he is adequately covered). When that sudden heart fear arises, you want and need a doctor fast.

Does your doctor keep his appointments? If I had a doctor who kept me waiting for hours in his outer office (or in one of his inner cubicles) time and again, I'd go scouting for another man who was aware that when you rob a man of his precious time, you rob him of more than his wallet. Being too busy is no excuse. A good doctor should not make more appointments than he can handle. He must plan to treat all of his patients efficiently.

Has he got a sense of humor? That is an important ingredient. If I were flat on my back for weeks, I'd hate to be greeted by a grumpy, cantankerous doctor every day.

Is the doctor willing to discuss fees and other expenses? I'd suspect a fellow who reared up on his hind legs when money was mentioned before an operation, delivery, or a long course of treatments. Financial worries compound the problems of the sick. The understanding physician will sit down with you and give you an adequate summary of the expenses involved. But remember what John Webster said, "Gold that buys health can never be ill spent."

If I were concerned about my heart, I'd want my doctor to have most or all of the attributes I have listed. Call such a man a saint if you prefer. I call him just a good doctor. If you have one like him, cherish him.

One patient said, "I think I have a very good doctor except that he has one failing—he doesn't give me a chance to talk. I know he is busy, but a patient expects at least a little time in the consulting room. The trouble is that he won't listen."

I have said it is important that your doctor have "big ears." He must realize that listening to his patient is perhaps one of the most important elements of the visit. Sometimes it is more important than the physical examination itself.

For example, often buried somewhere in the patient's story of his illness and complaints is the key that unlocks the apparently unyielding door to a correct diagnosis.

Suppose you have been bothered by stomach pains. The doctor orders a gastro-intestinal series of X rays. These prove negative. If he had heard you say that the pains are worse on an empty stomach and that a little milk makes them disappear like magic, he would not dismiss the possibility of a duodenal ulcer until he had made further investigation.

Or you say, "I have stomach pains only when I lie down to go to sleep, especially after a heavy meal. I like to lie flat and don't use any pillow." The expert diagnostician (and he is expert in direct ratio to the size of his ears) would immediately take measures to determine whether or not you have a diaphragmatic (hiatal) hernia. If he had missed these apparently innocuous words, he might have overlooked the true diagnosis.

37

One patient went to his doctor complaining of severe pain in his left wrist. He had had it for months and it was getting worse. "I never get it when I'm resting, only when I walk fast or get excited," he said.

If his doctor had not listened he might easily have overlooked the true diagnosis. Instead of looking for arthritis or sprain or something else, his mind focused on the words "only when I walk fast or get excited."

Although the typical story of the anginal patient is that he suffers pain or other distress under his chest, which extends down one or both arms on exertion, the doctor decided to investigate this atypical story. Unusual as it was, it turned out to be angina pectoris. If the doctor hadn't listened he would have erred in his diagnosis.

The good salesman knows when it is "listening time"; so does the smart housewife when her troubled husband comes home; so does the doctor when confronted with the anxious patient; so does the auto mechanic when your car needs attention.

I recently returned from a garage where my car was repaired by a mechanic who fancied himself a diagnostician. When I stopped by, I told him that something was wrong with my brakes. They seemed to work most of the time but occasionally they would completely fail. I told him I was fortunate that I hadn't had a bad accident. I had checked on my brake-fluid level. It was not quite full, so the gas attendant had added some.

"Did that make any difference in the brake action?" asked the mechanic. I told him it hadn't.

"Then I know what the diagnosis is," he said. "It's in your master cylinder. I can swear that's the trouble before I lift the hood. You know, if more mechanics listened carefully as people told their own story in their own way, they'd find the trouble without having to lift the hood."

38

He was right. I was there when he took down the master cylinder. He replaced a few worn parts, cleaned the cylinder, and the brakes worked like new.

I stood there while he repaired it, and all the while he kept on repeating, "If only mechanics would listen carefully, they wouldn't have to go messing around looking for the trouble. The history would tell them before they laid a hand on the car."

I have been tooting that horn for many years. I keep saying that doctors should find the time to listen and patients should come right out with a complete confession about what has been bothering them.

In so many cases a diagnosis of imaginary heart trouble is missed completely because of insufficient listening time. And in others, much unnecessary time is spent in the hospital or in taking laboratory tests in a futile attempt to make the diagnosis. A simple, history-taking session might have furnished the apparently elusive clues.

Here is a common complaint: "I'm afraid to open my mouth in my doctor's office. Whenever I ask him a question he looks at me as if I were a child in kindergarten speaking out of turn. Is he right or am I?"

Do you have an iron-bound contract? Is it impossible for you to dissolve your relationship? I doubt it. No doctor is *my* doctor. No patient is *my* patient. Neither owns the other. Free choice of doctor presupposes the free choice to engage someone else.

Personally, I wouldn't go to a physician who would shut me up. I might as well get my advice entirely out of a home medical adviser.

I recall one woman who could take it no longer. She told me about her experience at a party I attended several months ago.

"Year after year," she said, "I went to this doctor who

has such a fine reputation. Not only didn't he let me speak, but he hardly said a word after he had examined me. If I needed a new diet he handed me a printed sheet. If I needed medicine he handed me a prescription and only said, 'Take this as directed.' Nothing else.

"One week when he was out of town on his first vacation in many years, I visited another doctor. I couldn't believe what occurred. For at least half an hour this kindly man asked me questions and sat patiently as I answered. For the first time in my life, I felt I had a friend as well as a doctor. I never went back to the first man."

My reply was to agree that she had done the right thing.

Ordinarily I don't recommend doctor-changing. But I rarely hesitate to say try someone else when the patient complains "he is afraid to open his mouth" in his doctor's office. History-taking is one of the most important ways of tracking down the cause of illness. Any doctor who disabuses his position to shut off his patient cannot be an efficient and competent practitioner, no matter how many diplomas decorate his office walls.

Keep remembering that the doctor–patient relationship is a partnership. Refuse to be a silent partner if you value your health and life. Refuse to be "put down" in your doctor's presence if you worry about your heart. I can't understand why so many otherwise forthright people become so hesitant in the presence of a physician. Part of the answer, I suppose, is that when one's health and life teeter in the balance it is a human reaction to become flustered and unnaturally apprehensive.

On the other hand, some patients become irritable and incensed when the doctor fires probing questions at them. Instead of appreciating his need to take a full history, they resent it.

I remind such patients, "It is your health and your life.

It is your present and your future. But remember that your past is important, too. Your doctor, if he is thorough, patient and helpful, must be intensely curious about your past." Nevertheless some imaginary heart patients react like the following indignant letter writer, a woman in Milwaukee who was annoyed by her doctor's questions during a visit to his office:

> I was never so ashamed. I think my doctor went too far. Before he even laid a hand on me, he began asking me the most embarrassing questions. He wanted to know if there was any history in my family of tuberculosis, syphilis, or insanity. He asked me if I loved my husband; if my husband loved me. How was our sex life? Did we love our children? Did our children love us? Is my husband an alcoholic? What about our financial condition? Are we worried about it? Do I overeat? Do I have what I consider bad habits? He kept on like this for at least a half hour. Now wouldn't you think that a doctor would realize that his patients are sensitive and not ask so many personal questions?

The answer, of course, is that a complete history is a necessary part of the investigation. Not to obtain one is as fruitless and inefficient as a detective refusing to run down clues.

I have heard people express the opinion that some lawyers should be hung, that some businessmen should go bankrupt, that some doctors should drop dead. Psychiatrists state that there is much venom in the human spirit. Sometimes we get so mad, child and adult, that we wish (and live with the guilt for a while) the worst on our own loved ones. Therefore, it is not surprising to receive an occasional letter which blasts doctors:

> You continually ask the patient to "trust your doc-

41

tor." Try being a layman for a while and see your trust go down the drain. I've had a good deal of illness in my life, and I'm becoming an expert on doctors.

The first item that ruined the medical man was the discovery of "psychosomatic illness." This has become the lazy doctor's crutch for brushing off his patients. Even if he does not use the words, he plainly indicates by his actions that he thinks the problems are "psychosomatic." The average doctor today treats all patients who aren't carried in with bleeding wounds as psychosomatic patients.

Doctors have been so trained that when you ask a question, you get an answer in gobbledegook. Ask for an explanation and it takes a medical dictionary to understand the jargon. Protest about treatment which isn't working and you're told you don't know what you're talking about.

If you're five minutes late for an appointment you're charged for the appointment and told to make another one by the receptionist. Be five minutes early and you wait an hour. And it isn't only emergencies that cause the delay. Often the emergency is in the discussion of last Wednesday's golf game with the dentist across the hall.

American medicine screams (and I use the term advisedly) that it is the best medical care in the world. But why must almost all doctors adopt such a superior, patronizing attitude toward their patients? I do not go to see my doctor unless something is wrong with my heart and I dislike being told it is in my head. What do you think?

Here is how I answered the letter:

In your present state of mind, anything I say will be held against me. After all, you mustn't forget that I am a physician, too. When you berate "almost all" doctors, how superior must I be not to consider myself included, too? Nevertheless, I have always tried to be impartial—even if it hurts.

If you have been a regular reader of my column during the past fifteen years or so, undoubtedly you recall many dissertations (and many letters reprinted similar to yours) which did not hesitate to expose the profession to just criticism.

I, myself, have castigated some medical men for practicing quackery, for overcharging, for acting like little gods, for not making emergency calls, for keeping people waiting for hours in their offices.

However, here is where we differ; you say "almost all" doctors are like that. I say that very few doctors are like that. It seems it has been your bad luck to encounter one or more doctors with all these faults rolled up into one. It is for such reasons that I suggest (as I have previously) that patients should not hesitate to try another doctor or two until they find the "right one." You may be wondrously surprised to find a compassionate human being with an M.D. after his name who really cares. Most doctors do.

The good doctor is aware that the terror of the man with imaginary heart trouble is real, just as real as the terror of the sleeping child who wakes and runs from an *imaginary* witch in his dreams to the comfort of his parents' bed. This doctor knows that the frightened patient needs comfort and reassurance as does the child. And the anxious heart patient must believe in his doctor as the child does in his father or mother.

What is the doctor's job? Most important, it is to convince you that your heart is normal. And a hard job it often is. He can accomplish this by relieving your symptoms, or at least improving them. And he cannot do it simply by patting you on the back and saying, "Oh, forget it. There's nothing wrong. You have nothing to worry about." He may sometimes need to prescribe medicine, but he will always find it essential to take a full history, do a complete physical examination, and patiently explain the origin (and mechanics) of your symptoms.

In other words, for proper, effective management the competent physician will always call on these old reliables: his brain to think; his heart to sympathize and understand; attentive ears for good listening, and a tongue to explain, comfort, and outline treatment,

Before making a positive diagnosis of imaginary heart trouble (which is really a diagnosis of emotional stress rather than of disease) your physician must rule out organic heart disease. Having accomplished this, he settles down to ferret out the basic cause of your symptoms. At times, as I mentioned previously, he may seem to be an overly embarrassing and curious cuss as he prods you with personal questions. Nevertheless, these are essential.

If your imaginary heart condition is mild, your doctor may help you very easily. If your fear is more deeply imbedded, he might call in a cardiologist for advice and reassurance. Where symptoms are stubborn—and defy the regular attending physicians—the help of a psychiatrist may solve the riddle.

Keep remembering what Dr. William Menninger said: "No one, no matter how calm and complacent, is immune to psychoneurosis if the emotional strains get tough enough."

What greater proof is needed than the tension-produced breakdowns during World War I when the battle strains got too tough? The doctors called the condition DAH or "disordered action of the heart," when boys with healthy hearts complained of shortness of breath, of pain, palpitation, nervousness, fatigue, sweating, and anxiety. Later it was called "neurocirculatory asthenia." Now we commonly label it "anxiety neurosis."

But there were other observers who knew about it long before modern cardiology came upon the scene. In 1628, the year that brilliant Dr. William Harvey published his findings about the blood circulation, he also emphasized the effect of the mind upon the heart. He said, "Every affection of the mind that is attended with either pain or pleasure, hope or fear, is the cause of an agitation whose influence extends to the heart."

See how his basic truth affects us all today.

The daily reiteration of heart-disease deaths in newspapers often becomes a cumulative force that plants fear in abnormally introspective individuals. More people have become heart-conscious during the years since President Eisenhower's heart attacks than ever before. The public awareness of his courage while ill has saved the lives of thousands of Americans, but has left many abnormally fearful about their hearts.

Then there are the front-page headlines and stories about the new daring heart-transplant operations and other forms of cardiac surgery. And let us not forget the actual televised pictures of the beating heart under the knife! Many an absorbed viewer has confessed that he came away "heart-conscious" after witnessing in his own den a television heart operation.

How about the Heart Fund drive? Any cardiologist will tell you that the annual February Heart Campaign is the spur that invariably fills his appointment books for weeks. Anxious people come for reassurance. I recall complimenting a busy executive on his good sense in coming in for yearly physical checkups.

"Frankly, I can't take the credit," he said. "The annual heart drive scares me into doing what's good for me."

45

We should all be thankful for such heart publicity. I have often told patients, and it bears repetition, "I'd rather you turn out to be a live, fully informed hypochondriac who lives to be 80, than to remain a medically uninformed, falsely secure, superoptimist who is shuffled off at 40."

Most doctors are beginning to realize that patients anxious about their heart can be thrown into a dither of uncertainty, fear, and chronic anxiety in many ways. Therefore, we try to handle all patients tactfully. We try to be careful about what we do, what we say—and how we do it and say it. Otherwise, we ourselves may implant heart fear in patients.

For example, many a well-adjusted man or woman becomes heart-conscious after being rejected by an insurance examiner. Offhanded remarks such as "You have a murmur" or "Your pressure's much too high" or "Better get to your doctor for an examination—quick" are inciting factors for the impressionable. But insurance examiners are not alone to blame. We practicing physicians must plead guilty to causing much imaginary heart trouble. For example, consider iatrogenic heart disease:

Dr. G. Gillespie wrote in the *British Medical Journal:* "There is a chapter omitted from medical books which might be headed iatrogenic disease; that is to say, disease produced by doctors."

Consider the manner in which some doctors explain the presence of organic disease: "You have a big leak." "Keep this up and you're likely to drop dead." "The insides of your coronary arteries are closing up like a rusty pipe." These are only a few of the many variations on a similar horrid theme.

Much, of course, depends on the physician. He should be aware that he must interest himself in the patient with a heart problem *as a person* rather than *as a case*. The tactful practitioner is on constant guard against subdued cluckings and raised eyebrows when taking a blood pressure reading or when making a stethoscopic examination.

He doesn't mention a murmur when it is functional and harmless. He doesn't say, "Your murmur is borderline." He doesn't say, "Your electrocardiogram is borderline." (Either it *is* normal or it *isn't*.)

Novelist Ben Ames Williams once published an article in the *New England Journal of Medicine* (in the issue of October 11, 1945) titled "The Greeks Had a Word for It." Five months before its publication, he had delivered it as a speech at the George W. Gay Lecture on Medical Ethics at Harvard Medical School.

I recommend it as reading for lay as well as medical audiences. It has a depth of understanding suitable for the mind of any reader. Here are some salient quotations from it:

> You will decide how you will treat his [the patient's] mind before you decide how you will treat his body. The prospect of summoning a doctor, for himself or for one of his family, frightens almost every layman.
>
> I suspect that every medical school should have a course of lectures given by patients! Certainly any doctor after having once been ill himself is a better doctor afterwards.
>
> The lesson that every doctor most needs to learn is that his patients are afraid.
>
> The wise doctor will remember that it may be quite as easy to make a well person sick as to make a sick person well.
>
> The most dangerous drug you can administer to your patient is fear.
>
> It is the hard lot of the doctor to know that in the end he is always defeated; his victories at best are temporary. Death he can never finally conquer. But

death's ally is fear, and this ally the doctor can defeat. Let him help the patient to conquer fear.

More and more, the doctor should be less and less the cause of imaginary heart trouble. This is so because he should realize that the outwardly calm patient may be nervous "inside."

As Dr. Andrew D. Hart wrote in the *Journal of the American Medical Association:*

> Patients with psychosomatic disease may show little or no evidence of emotional instability. The outward tension phenomena commonly associated with neurotic disposition and with psychoneuroses are often absent.

I recall two patients, of many, who illustrate that it is an important part of the doctor's job to handle patients with care.

One was a popular minister whose sermons brought in his parishioners and kept them awake. He was a confident, skillful, and learned speaker. He had been a patient of mine for years.

While on vacation he complained of chest pain. He consulted a physician in a neighboring town who told him that he had had a questionable coronary attack. But the ECG's were negative, so he discharged him. But that was not all. In attempting to warn the minister of possible future trouble, he was too forceful in his admonition.

When he returned home, this terribly apprehensive patient told me: "You would think doctors should show more sense. I went to one of the best last week when I had this so-called attack during my vacation. After his examination he showed me pictures of blocked-off coronaries, ruptured hearts, and other scary things out of a big medical book, trying to impress me to be alert. When he finished he said, 'That's the kind of trouble you're headed for if you're not careful.' I almost fainted right there—and I've been scared to death of my heart ever since."

About a week after he returned, he called me at home and asked if I would do him a favor. He had suddenly lost all confidence in himself. He admitted that he was actually afraid to face his congregation the following night.

"Would you find time," he said, "to come and sit in the front row where I can see you while I deliver the sermon? Knowing you are there will give me the confidence to carry on."

For the next four Sundays I sat there, in full view, occasionally nodding my head and smiling reassuringly as he spoke. I watched him as he courageously fought off his fears. He used his handkerchief quite often to wipe away the perspiration on his forehead. I doubt that any other of his parishioners even suspected the strength of will evinced by his determination to face his congregation. Not until a few months later did his former confidence return in full.

The second patient I recall, and shall never forget, was the wife of a prominent businessman. One day she had an attack of "acute indigestion." A doctor called in emergency diagnosed it as a coronary attack. He told her she'd have to remain in bed for at least two months. Dissatisfied with his treatment at the end of a week, she discharged him and called me.

Electrocardiograms and other tests were negative at the end of two weeks. I told her she did not have coronary trouble and that she could get right out of bed. It took much convincing to win her compliance. She was overweight, had a round, bright face, and a lower lip with a tendency to tremble when she talked about herself.

X rays later showed she had a gall bladder filled with stones, which had probably been the reason for her acute indigestion. The subsequent operation was uneventful and she recovered nicely. But there remained a residue of fear. She was still not convinced that her heart was all right.

Then she committed the not uncommon patient-sin of getting another unannounced medical opinion while under the care of a physician. This was her story when she next visited my office:

"You know I have all the confidence in the world in you. But I must admit that I have been so scared about my heart that I sought out another opinion. I went to Dr. —, who you know is one of the best heart specialists in the East. He examined me and said that although I have no definite coronary disease, I have arteriosclerosis.

"I asked him what that meant. Would I have coronary trouble later? I asked him what would happen if one coronary artery got blocked off.

"He took out a book and showed me a blocked-off coronary. Suppose that happened to me, I asked him again? What might happen if the other one got blocked off, too?

"All he did was shrug his shoulders, raise his eyebrows and say, 'Nothing, I suppose, except your family would have to put a call in to the undertaker.' "

Her lip trembled as never before. She fidgeted in her chair. The shine of panic filled her eyes. She began to cry. I did all I could to reassure her, not realizing that for the next twenty-five years I would still be trying to obliterate from her mind what might happen if one or both of her coronary arteries were shut off. She died at the age of seventy-two. The cause? A coronary attack!

Before she died she was more composed than she had ever been, and there was an accusing gleam in her eyes when she looked at me. It was as if she was saying, "See, doctor, I was right. I might have had coronary trouble all the time." (The thousand deaths that she had died during all those years were more painful and worrisome to her than her first, actual attack of heart disease.)

A patient deserves to know the truth. You cannot adequately treat a cardiac without his full cooperation. Withholding the truth for fear of alarming the patient negates any potential benefits of examination and prescribed treatment.

Most patients want to know the truth even though they do not welcome unfavorable verdicts. It is at this point in the telling that the experience, sympathy, and tactfulness of the physician count for so much. We doctors treat human beings, each a potential storehouse of fear. A mite of understanding and tact can prevent undue anxiety. Once the dread of heart disease becomes imbedded, ten tactful physicians may have difficulty in neutralizing it.

Dr. J. A. Oille in the *Canadian Medical Journal* provides some interesting statistics:

> Almost sixty percent of patients who consult a cardiac specialist are suffering from either an exaggerated or a wholly unnecessary anxiety about their hearts, arising from suggestion and not based on reason, most suggestions following the careless or ill-considered remarks of doctors.

Dr. Walter Alvarez has put it well: "The victim may suddenly, at any time of the day or night, feel jittery or ill—with the heart racing or missing beats. It is well for physicians to remember that there are such syndromes, that they are common, and that they are caused by erratic nerves or an erratic brain which is playing tricks with a perfectly normal heart."

Your doctor will be expected to be aware of your in-

51

tense anxiety. He has a job to do. Briefly here is your doctor's job:

1. He will not "laugh off" your fears and dismiss you with a perfunctory "forget it" and a pat on the back.

2. He will be sympathetic and take a complete, unhurried history as he listens to your complaints.

3. He will, nevertheless, use all modern diagnostic tools at his command: complete physical examination, fluoroscopic and X-ray surveys, electrocardiograms, and the indicated laboratory tests.

4. Having completed his investigation he will tell you the *truth*. Either you *have* heart disease or you do not.

5. If the diagnosis is real heart disease, you can be thankful it was discovered early. Your doctor will prescribe medicines or surgery, and a new way of life that will prolong your years.

6. If the diagnosis is imaginary heart trouble, he will give you reassurance and the necessary medications to overcome your discomforts and fears.

What better way to sum up the doctor's job than by quoting the words of B. Kresky, M.D., as they appeared in an article written for the American Heart Association:

If a patient has a cardiac neurosis, a positive explanation is in order that there is no heart disease; that there need not be any limitation of activity; that the symptoms are not referable to the heart. . . .

The patient must be advised that some of his complaints are due to anxiety about his heart and conflicts in his life situation rather than to a cardiac lesion. By reassurance and guidance, the physician can often do much to allay anxiety and help the patient make a more comfortable adjustment.

Now that you have learned what to expect from your

doctor and from yourself, let us turn to tips on how to overcome your anxiety about your heart.

Are you especially concerned when your heart begins to skip? Are you "sure" the pain in your left chest spells heart disease and impending doom? Are you still worried about that murmur you first heard about when you were a child many years ago? Are your friends correct in saying your protracted fatigue is most likely due to a failing heart? Are you still uncertain about the results of your electrocardiographic examination?

From these and similar seeds of doubt and fear does the large tree of anxiety grow.

I intend to show you how to live with yourself, with your associates, with your family and friends as a well-integrated individual should. Not in unnatural bravado, but not in unnatural fear, either.

PART II

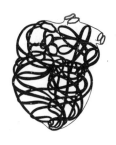

WHAT YOU CAN DO
FOR "HEART TROUBLE"

4.

WHEN YOUR HEART SKIPS, AND JUMPS, AND "RUNS AWAY"

Among the worst sufferers from heart trouble are those who do not have heart disease. Although it is true that millions of Americans do have real heart disease, at least 15 million of us think we have—but actually do not. Our heart symptoms may be *real* but our disease is *imaginary*.

Scores of anxious patients have asked me, "What do you mean when you say 'imaginary heart trouble'? That we are just imagining things when the heart begins to skip? That we just imagine we are scared to death that the heart will never start beating again after it skips? Take it from one who admits he is frightened about it all. These skips are more than in the mind. I don't just imagine them!"

When I say "imaginary" I don't say so in any derogatory sense. Patients do not imagine the skips. They are there. But what they are imagining is that their heart is sick or weak or diseased when it isn't.

I have treated thousands of people who experienced skips, yet had normal hearts. These skips were functional and had nothing to do with organic heart disease. Yet, I had difficulty convincing these frightened people that the skips would not shorten their lives.

Fortunately, some men and women are more optimistic by nature, and take their skips in stride. For example, consider this patient who has had heart skips since he was in his twenties. His letter is a refreshingly cheerful document:

> My goodness, all these young people of thirty-five and forty worrying whether or not they'll live long enough to grow old. Here, I'm over seventy, and have had these skips for almost a lifetime.
>
> I've never let them frighten me. Just went right along living, doing things everybody else did, and trusted in the Lord. When my doctor said my heart was all right, I took him at his word. I feel fine and life is great.
>
> I ran into one of these frightened people the other day. He was telling me it was close to the end because he had been noticing a few heart skips for the past week. Although his doctor took electrocardiograms and all the rest, and gave him a good bill of health, he was bemoaning the fact that he was only forty-two and didn't want to die so young.
>
> I felt like telling him the story of the old boy who drank and smoked and chased women all his life— died at the age of eighty-four—and when he was three days dead, the old fellow looked better than this frightened soul did right now. But he was much bigger than me, so I kept quiet.
>
> My own doctor keeps telling me I check out fine in my annual exams and I believe him, leave the office and forget the skips when they come. In fact, I tell my doctor when he's overdoing by getting too fat. He's thinking of hiring me as his medical adviser. There's one hitch—I don't know a damn thing about medicine.

But I have noticed that most people are more or less "uptight" about themselves until they're about sixty. After that, they tend to relax and ask themselves what all the fussin' and the frettin' was about! Not all of them, of course, but the sensible ones. It's too bad that some frightened people are taking medicines for diseases that haven't even been discovered yet.

Personally, I figure if it can't be cured with a bourbon and ginger ale once in a while, it can't be cured.

Cheerfully yours, Frank M.

I have experienced heart skips myself. Although I know that they are not life-shortening, I agree that waiting for the next heart beat to come through can seem like an interminably long time. But invariably it does occur. All I am saying is believe your doctor if he says your heart is all right. Don't borrow trouble that isn't there.

Have you ever felt your heart skip a beat? Sometimes it feels like a sudden slap in the chest; others say it is as if "something seems to turn over in the throat." I do not expect a few words of reassurance to enable an anxious patient to immediately overcome deep-seated emotion. Yet, I think you should know the ABC's of the anatomical and physiological nature of skipped beats (extrasystoles —often also called premature contractions).

The human body is the first wonder of the world. Made of a network of bones (206), muscles (639), and nerves and blood vessels (millions), it is the most efficient organism ever created. At the center of the vortex of movement, intelligence, and emotion is one bundle of muscles called the heart. It differs from all other muscles in that the heart muscle fibers are not separated into sheaths or bundles as are ordinary skeletal muscle fibers. Instead, these fibers are joined into a continuous network.

There are three main kinds of muscle in the body.

59

(1) Striped or skeletal muscle, known as voluntary muscle, is attached to some part of the skeleton. The brain sends down signals for such muscles to contract, and each tiny muscle fiber reacts quickly to these orders.

(2) Smooth muscle fibers are part of the involuntary muscle system over which you have no control. They receive their signals from a special nerve network called the autonomic nervous system. They function so automatically we are seldom aware of their work. Unlike skeletal muscles, smooth muscle contracts slowly and rhythmically—otherwise our stomach and intestines would forever be in cramps.

(3) Heart muscle, or cardiac muscle, is the type called striated muscle and it powers the most efficient pump in existence. The heart is the most wondrous of all muscles, about the size of your fist. It begins to beat months before you are born and continues until you die.

With only a fraction of a second's rest following each beat, it pumps blood 100,000 times a day, 40 million times a year. It pumps it through the arteries at forty miles an hour so that the blood can reach the tiny blood capillaries in which it slows down to a speed of only one inch a minute.

Each time the heart contracts, it ejects as much as three ounces of blood from each ventricle. This all adds up in twenty-four hours of its work to pumping as much as 2,000 gallons of blood a day (equivalent to lifting twelve tons a distance of one foot).

All this happens while you are at rest. When called upon by an emergency or by hard work, the heart can augment its ordinary output ten to twelve times by increasing the amount of blood ejected at each stroke and by increasing its rate. For example, under strenuous exercise the heart's output increases from a resting level of

60

five to six quarts a minute to between nineteen and thirty-seven quarts. You will admit that this is evidence of almost unlimited capacity to adjust to all conditions.

But where does all this forceful contraction begin? We call it the sino-auricular node, and it is situated in the right auricle (the right upper chamber of the heart). The electrical impulse spreads from this area quickly down into the ventricles (lower chambers), which respond with the normal heart contractions. Normally, we are unaware of the heart's beat. Only when the heart muscle becomes so irritable that all beats do not originate in the sino-auricular node do we realize that something "different" is happening.

You will suddenly become aware that your heart beat is not following its normal sequence. Something has happened to throw it out of rhythm. There has been a sudden premature contraction which originates elsewhere. The formerly silent beats make themselves known to you by slapping your chest, "turning over in your throat." Since there is a lengthy pause after each extrasystole or premature contraction, we think the next beat may never come.

We call it a skipped beat. With it emerges awareness of life—and death. Anxiety has stalked in with its train of sleeplessness, worry, fatigue, and loss of interest in many former activities. A housewife consulted me recently about her specific problem. She was tense and irritable during the visit and spoke with a great sense of urgency.

"I have a complaint and I do hope you can give me an answer for it. I have terrible, odd feelings in the middle of my chest as often as four or five times a day.

"When I have them, they last only for a second or two. But they cut off my breathing temporarily. Even after it is over, my heart beats real hard; not fast, but real hard for a few beats.

"There is no pain involved whatever. At times I have

61

put my finger on my pulse at the wrist when I get these spells and I don't feel any movement. Right after it, I feel the pulse beat again.

"When I get these awful feelings I am quite tired for a while afterward. It is a kind of rolling and fluttering feeling. I really can't explain it, but I hope I have told you enough for you to tell me what it is and what to do about it. I am afraid it is my heart. I am thirty-seven years old and have eight children, if that will help you any. My father died of a heart attack. His mother and sister died of strokes and my cousin on his side recently suffered a stroke."

When she finished her recital, she sat back in her chair seemingly exhausted, her cheeks pale and drawn, her eyes haggard. I gave her an examination, ran her through a series of tests including X rays, electrocardiogram, blood pressure readings, and I came to the conclusion that she was having heart skips, a common complaint that frightens thousands of people into thinking they have heart disease even though their hearts are normal—especially those who have a family history of heart disease and stroke, and who translate their own discomforts into a potentially serious disability. Fortunately, I was able to convince her, with proper medication and reassurance, that her heart was normal.

Here is a letter I received several months ago from a concerned reader:

> I have palpitation of the heart. Is it serious enough to kill or is there some simple remedy for it? It only bothers me at night. I just can't go to sleep. I roll and toss from side to side, and it becomes worse when I am on my back.
>
> During the past two years, I have had three electro-

cardiograms and my doctor says, I have nothing to worry about. I go to bed between 8:30 and 9:00 every night. These spells sometimes last all night and I get very little sleep.

My doctor does not give me a definite answer, good or bad. I'm seventy years old and do part-time jobs. All day I just feel grand. I know there must be something wrong somewhere.

In this instance, I happened to know another cardiologist in the patient's area and I suggested he visit him. My doctor friend ran his own independent tests and subsequently prescribed some quinidine. Happily, these pills quickly eliminated the man's heart skips.

Whenever you are in doubt about any illness, especially if heart disease is the question mark, do not hesitate to ask for a consultation if your doctor seems to be hedging. Where heart disease is involved, the patient deserves to know the entire truth. The doctor's reply should be unequivocal. Patients can't live in comfort on evasive answers to their questions about the heart.

Skipped beats are not the only cause of heart awareness in those with strong hearts. Another fairly common symptom is the sudden jump or large beat that can interrupt the rhythmic pattern of contractions in the heart.

Still another disagreeable symptom is the racing or runaway heart. Suddenly the heart increases its normal velocity like the sprinter who catapults off his starting blocks. It may suddenly race at 180 to 220 (or more) beats per minute. Here, for example, is a letter received recently from such a patient:

> I wonder if you can suggest what might be the cause of a peculiar thing that happened to me yesterday afternoon. I worked in the office until noon as usual on Sat-

63

urday, had a light lunch, then washed my car which is a compact and really no problem. I use a brush attach- ed to the hose, and rub with the brush as the water comes out.

I felt a little tired while holding the hose in an awk- ward position, and maybe my heart beat a little faster, which I thought understandable under the circumstan- ces. One gets "soft" in winter. I finished the job, and came inside the house and started sorting the clean laundry, sheets, towels spread out on the bed. It called for a tiny bit of stooping, but nothing unusual.

While doing this, my heart suddenly began beating very hard indeed, with a body-shaking thump, thump. A little alarmed, I decided to sit down. The thumping kept on for at least five minutes, then suddenly settled down to normal and I got up and finished the job.

There have been a few occasions in the past (I'm sure they occur to everyone) when my heart has beat hard suddenly for a couple of beats, but this was the first time it lasted so long. It was such a hard, rhythmic thumping that it veritably shook my frame. It seemed to be in the middle of my chest and not on the left side.

I had no difficulty in breathing whatsoever, and ab- solutely no pain. I felt fine the whole time, but it was such an upheaval that it was a little tiring. Perhaps for a tiny moment I felt a little bit nauseated.

I've been fine ever since. I'll be sixty-three in May, enjoy excellent health, weigh 152 and am five feet nine inches tall. I get an annual physical checkup by a most reputable doctor and take all the usual tests. I intend to mention it to my doctor when I see him again. Mean- while, I thought I'd write to you for an explanation. It certainly was, to me, a strange occurrence.

You will note how this patient with apparent paroxysmal tachycardia reacted to this attack of rapid heart action. Calmly, with no apprehension: "I intend to mention it to my doctor when I see him again." Not everyone accepts sudden runaway beats with such equanimity. Most people become frightened and remain that way, even after the heart has returned to its normal rhythm.

Admittedly, it is strange and often terrifying to have a quietly beating heart suddenly race as if it had been whipped by some sadistic, driving force. There are no specific known causes for these rapid beats that originate outside the normal pacemaker of the heart—in some irritable portion of the heart muscle.

In most patients the heart races for only a few beats; in others the rapid action may endure for hours or even days. Such rapid action does not endanger the individual's life, and can be reverted to a normal rate by drugs and other available methods to slow the heart.

Another patient wrote me a letter, describing her symptoms in this fashion:

> I have what is called tachycardia of the heart. I am just about ready to have a nervous breakdown from worrying. Every time I have such an attack I think I am going to die. I smother and have a nervous chill. I keep wondering about my heart even though I have been to two good doctors who have assured me that my heart is normal and I have nothing to worry about.
>
> Sometimes I have two or three attacks a week. Every time I have a palpitation in my chest, I think I am going to have another spell. I had my first attack of runaway heart about ten months ago. I almost passed out at first, but it stops suddenly just like it begins.
>
> I worry all the time. I am in my forties. I have a wonderful husband and three lovely children. I can't enjoy them because I worry so much I may suddenly have to leave them. I know I'll feel better if I hear from you. Gratefully, Mrs. Charles S.

I replied to this greatly concerned woman as follows:

You say you know you will feel better when you hear from me. Fine. However, all I can do is put together a few pieces of the puzzle (only your own doctors can be certain of the true diagnosis). They say you have no actual heart disease so I must guess that your rapid heart action is due to episodes of what we call paroxysmal tachycardia. This regular, rapid heart action can occur (as they say) in normal hearts.

I recall an incident in which a collegue took drastic steps to overcome a similar fear in a patient. The man was in an attack of paroxysmal tachycardia and was fearful he was going to die. He was a good swimmer, so the doctor set out to relieve his mind of his fears.

He took him out to a neighboring lake, told the man to put on his swimsuit, got into a rowboat himself, and followed him in a mile swim.

When his patient reached shore alive, heart still pumping away merrily, he looked at his doctor and said, "You've made your point. I'll never be scared when these attacks come on again."

I am not suggesting the water treatment for you, but I hoped the anecdote will reassure you that the most frightening hops, skips and jumps and runaway beats can occur in hearts which are not the seat of actual disease. Some hearts, for one reason or another (sometimes emotional) act up like skittish colts. They jump all over the place for a while. In view of your own doctors' reassurance, keep remembering that your heart is all right.

Irregularity of the heart in normal hearts is not uncommon. As H. M. Marvin, M.D., has put it:

In a fairly large percentage of healthy people the heart does not beat with absolute regularity. Even if the rate per minute remains almost unchanged, there may be variations in its rhythm. Most of the irregularities that occur in normal people are of no importance whatever, but some of them may cause slight discomfort.

If the person is aware of the irregularity, he may develop mild anxiety because of the belief it necessarily indicates heart disease. . . . Most experienced doctors believe that premature beats occur at times in all people. Certainly they are present in most, even during periods of apparently perfect health. . . .

Paroxysmal tachycardia does not injure the [normal] heart, does not lead to heart disease, does not threaten the life or future activities of the patient. (From *Your Heart,* A Handbook for Laymen, published by Doubleday and Co., 1960.)

It is simple to be some kind of philosopher on a full stomach; likewise, it may be easy to convince the patient whose heart is behaving, not skipping or running away with itself, that there is no reason for apprehension. However, the one undergoing the discomforts of heart skips or very rapid heart action is like the man with the empty stomach, it's difficult to make a philosopher of him.

"I'm scared to death," he says. "Don't just fill me with explanations. Do something! Or at least tell me what I can do while I'm having a heart attack." (You will note, he says, "heart attack," in spite of attempts to influence him against believing his heart is the seat of serious disease.)

Well, there are things to do.

For example, if you are having skips the thing to do may be *nothing.* Most people get over them without any treatment whatever. You may have the "cure" within your own grasp.

Perhaps you are too fat from overeating. You starve yourself at breakfast and lunch but make up for it at the evening meal. Then you stuff yourself. A sudden enlargement of the stomach can, in my experience, bring on heart irregularities in some patients.

If you fit into this category, try spacing your calories instead of taking them all in one evening dose.

Late on a Saturday night one November several years ago I received a hurry call. I had spent a pleasant afternoon at the Yale Bowl, watching a football game between Dartmouth and Yale. After taking in a movie later on and reading a few pages, I called it a day and turned in to sleep. Within a few minutes the phone rang. Picking up the receiver, I heard the voice of the twenty-three-year-old son of a neighbor of mine.

"Come quickly," he urged. "Mother is having a heart attack."

Since the family lived just around the corner, it wasn't long before I reached the house. Lights were on all over and the son was waiting for me at the door as I hurried up the front steps.

The mother lay in bed, eyes seeking mine for comfort, her forehead wet with perspiration. Although she was still fully dressed, I could see her heart pound rapidly. I loosened her dress so I could slip my stethoscope on her chest. Her heart rate was over 200 beats per minute.

She was a plump woman, at least fifty pounds overweight. A few weeks earlier during a visit to my office I had warned her to melt off some of that excess poundage.

Otherwise, she was a healthy woman. Undoubtedly she was now having an attack of paroxysmal tachycardia. It was her first attack. I learned that she and her son had been to the Yale game, too. They had visited members of the family while in New Haven. She had eaten "enough for four" because she had been so hungry.

There are three dramatic ways to stop an attack of paroxysmal tachycardia. The first two I tried were unsuccessful. One, I applied pressure to her eyeballs. Two, I pressed on one side of her neck in the carotid area (over the carotid artery). Then I tried on the other side. (Pressure should not be brought on both sides simultaneously. We want to slow the heart rate, not stop it entirely.)

Then I looked for a way to institute the third method of treatment. I wanted to induce vomiting. Sudden emptying of the stomach can bring a runaway heart to a sudden, screeching halt. On the night table I saw a blue feather with Y-A-L-E emblazoned on it. The family had brought it back from the game.

I grabbed it, asked the woman to open her mouth, tickled the back of her pharynx with it, and she quickly brought up the remains of her dinner. Her symptoms were relieved.

Suppose you are normal weight and are plagued by heart skips? Where else shall you look? Re-examine your habits. Do you smoke? How much? In so many patients with heart skips the irregularities have disappeared within days after cutting down (or out) the tobacco intake. Do you drink? How much? For some people, one martini or a jigger of scotch will act as a whip and send the heart off into capers.

Do the skips or rapid beats come on with extreme fatigue? With nervous tension? Then it is your job to neutralize these heart irritants in your susceptible muscle. Have you been suffering from insomnia? Then perhaps a sleeping pill prescribed by your physician will break up the vicious circle that produces your symptoms.

69

Tranquilizers often relax the anxious patient sufficiently so that his fears become shadowy outlines rather than actual menaces he can clearly see. I tell patients not to "be afraid" of taking them under the doctor's constant observation. They become "dope" only when the patient bootlegs these pills without the doctor's knowledge, increasing the dosage from week to week.

Quinidine has been a standby for years in the management of heart skips and other heart irregularities. Proper dosage is essential. Likewise, when digitalis is used to control heart irregularities. Another drug that is often successful is Pronestyl.

But most important of all is the need for reassurance —repeated as often as necessary. There must be no room for impatience in the doctor's office simply because the patient reiterates the fears he complained about weeks previously.

For example, I heard the following complaint from one woman week after week for at least a year. It was a typical case history I had heard hundreds of times from other patients. She was a forty-four-year-old housewife, overweight, with bulging eyes. She looked like a hyperthyroid patient but she wasn't.

She said: "I never worried about anything in my life like I do about my heart. Every night, before I finish reading and am ready to turn off my bed light, my heart suddenly turns over in my throat and thumps my chest. I keep thinking it's the end. I almost die of fright. Instead of calling my husband, I fight off the fear and finally fall asleep. I'm convinced my heart is beginning to give out." (She lived into her mid-seventies. Tranquilizers, quinidine, and reassurance had made life livable and joyful many years earlier.)

If I were asked the most important essential for re-

covery from imaginary heart trouble I would answer:
FAITH.

I recall one tiny woman who at last overcame her anxieties about her heart. I asked her how she had accomplished this seemingly impossible solution. She said what so many do: "First God; then the doctor."

I told her that she had left out one important factor: herself. Faith in the ultimate cure could only rise first from the depths of her own being.

She nodded her head in agreement, like a youngster accepting a compliment with self-consciousness, and said, "I guess you're right, Doctor."

5.

CHEST PAIN IS NOT INVARIABLY HEART PAIN

The daily challenge the physician must meet is correct diagnosis.

Unless your doctor makes the fitting diagnosis you, the patient, suffer for it. Therefore, as I have said in previous chapters, the two (or more) of you should pool all your information to help in coming to the right conclusion.

For example, consider coronary disease. We are always on guard against overlooking this diagnosis. As often happens where suspicion is uppermost, sometimes we point the finger at the innocent. Undoubtedly, thousands of patients labeled as having coronary disease do not have any trouble in these heart arteries.

Knowing this, we doctors try to make certain that the patient's chest pain or other discomfort may not be due to something outside the heart: gall bladder disease, pancreatitis, stomach ulcer, hiatal hernia, inflammation of the pleura (lung covering), bursitis, arthritis, shingles—which often simulate coronary pain.

Here, for example, is another condition that often makes a correct diagnosis difficult. It is frequently confused with serious heart or lung disease. A common name for it is "painful cartilage."

The patient comes in complaining of various degrees of chest discomfort. Sometimes it is worse on changing position or taking deep breaths. Even turning in bed at night can produce the pain in the chest. The patient lies rigid in fear, certain he is having a heart attack. But examination, laboratory tests, and electrocardiograms are negative. The diagnosis is definitely not that of coronary thrombosis.

The doctor presses over the front of the chest where ribs meet cartilage (called the costochondral junctions) and he discovers that the patient is extremely sensitive to pressure. By pressing here, the doctor is able to reproduce the patient's symptoms. We don't know what causes this condition (perhaps heavy work, perhaps sudden strain such as in severe coughing spells), but it is relieved often with heat applications, aspirin, and the use of a tight bandage or brassiere. Sometimes injections of cortisone help.

Dr. Maurice S. Rawlings of Chattanooga, Tennessee, writing in the periodical *Diseases of the Chest,* described fifty patients with this acute and chronic rib syndrome. He found that the most commonly affected area was in the second and third cartilage rib junctions on the left side of the chest.

The fear of heart disease is a natural phenomenon because everyone is aware that it is the number one killer. Therefore, anything which calls attention to the heart brings on, especially in overly nervous persons, an anxiety about the heart.

I recall a spirited, middle-aged, retired school teacher who had been working in her flower beds. It was her first exertion of this kind in months, and she spent hours at it. After she came in to have some tea, she suddenly suffered a pain in her chest on bending over to pick up a napkin from the floor. It lasted the rest of the afternoon and into the night.

When she lay flat, the pain was gone, but when she turned on her side it came back. At first she dismissed it as being some sort of muscle spasm. But when it persisted for more than a week, she became anxious about her heart. Yet, she thought it too silly to bother her doctor, since the pain was not so distressing now.

At last, after months of worry, she came to my office. She was suffering from "painful cartilage." A few aspirins a day and the use of a heat pad quickly cleared up her symptoms.

Fortunately, she was easily convinced that her heart was sound. She did not remain neurotically concerned that her coronary arteries were possibly the cause of the pain. She is only one example that all patients who fear heart disease do not continue to be anxious about themselves. An adequate explanation is sufficient to bring them back to normality.

Unfortunately, the "memory" of pain remains imbedded so deeply in the consciousness of some susceptible persons that it produces a revolution in their normal course of existence. They continue to live scared.

For example, consider the following case history, of a thirty-five-year-old man, married, part-owner of an automobile agency, the father of three children, and husband of a sweet wife.

"I want to live as long as I can, for my family and myself," he began as he took a chair across from my desk. He was a small man, of average weight for his age and well but conservatively dressed. "But here is my problem. I had some chest pains a few months ago which lasted only a few minutes. A doctor took one electrocardiogram and said he 'thought' but 'wasn't sure' that I had some abnormality.

"Although it wasn't a typical heart attack, he warned me that I'd have to live carefully and especially watch my diet to keep my blood cholesterol down to normal."

He paused a moment, his gray eyes fixed on my face. "I think I may have become too 'preventive-medicine-conscious.' Every living minute I ask myself if I am doing something which may make me real sick. At work, at home, while on vacation I keep saying to myself: 'Is this harmful?' Now, doctor, don't you think I'm overdoing it?" There was a faint, half-apologetic smile tugging at his thin mouth as he finished.

In effect, here is what I said to him: "Let me show you a mirror image and see if you recognize yourself. Seeing yourself as you see others may do more to give you a new philosophy of life than any preaching I may do on the subject.

"The other day a business man in his early forties said to me, 'I've become very coronary-conscious. Many of my pals and my own business partner have been struck down by a coronary attack. I'll tell you what I've done to prevent it from striking me. I used to have a big breakfast: a glass of orange juice, coffee, two cups with cream, three slices of buttered toast, oatmeal, two eggs, and a large side order of ham or bacon.

" 'About a year ago I cut out the eggs, ham, and bacon because I'd heard that too much cholesterol was bad. A few months later, I heard that even carbohydrates turn into cholesterol so I cut out the oatmeal, bread, and orange juice.

" 'That left only the cup or two of black coffee to give me a start in the morning. And just last week, I read that some doctors had discovered that coffee is instrumental in building up too much fat in the blood stream, too. So I cut that out.

" 'Now I go to work on an empty stomach. It's tough on a man who has been used to fortifying himself with a big, nourishing breakfast. I am famished by lunch time. I am sure my efficiency has been cut in half. What would you do?' "

"I told the patient that he was riding the pendulum of medical opinion and it was swinging him about too far. I reminded him we are not yet certain that cholesterol in foods is the potential death of all of us. It has not yet clearly been tied in as the direct cause of coronary thrombosis. Nor are we certain that carbohydrates or coffee are enemies of our arteries.

"Rather than live in unnecessary anxiety I suggest you live in moderation. I say this because your blood pressure is normal, your blood cholesterol is not elevated, you are not overweight, you have no diabetes, nor do you have a family history of artery disease. You don't smoke or overdrink and you try not to live in continual stress.

"In spite of what you have been hearing, there are still many healthy men of your age who need not restrict their intake of cholesterol-rich foods such as butter, eggs, ice cream, and fatty meats. I tell them to live a normal life. If they like a breakfast of ham and eggs they may have it. So is coffee all right and orange juice.

"I believe that a moderately large breakfast which consists of portions of fats, carbohydrates, and proteins is certainly better for a normal person than starving himself for a greater part of the day. Don't live as if you are already sick. You can overdo it. Pretty soon you will be afraid to cross the street after reading the latest auto accident statistics. Start living."

My thirty-five-year-old patient left the office a happy man. He returned to his former way of life and lived for many years without a rise in his cholesterol or any evidence of coronary disease. What was most important is that he lived without undue anxiety.

Often, it is the wife who makes a cholesterolophobe out of her healthy husband. Although I advise wives to "nag" their husbands into taking care of themselves when there is indisputable evidence of illness, there are times when they become unnecessarily concerned. For example, consider this letter received from an apprehensive wife:

> In thirty-two years of married life my husband has had only one physical examination—when he served in the Second World War! He is self-employed and reluctant to leave his business if only for a few hours.
>
> I am concerned mainly because he insists upon a breakfast of juice, two eggs, a large helping of cottage cheese, buttered toast and two cups of coffee with evaporated milk. Two or three times weekly he wants several pork sausages or bacon. He also helps himself to a large serving of ice cream before going to bed. I have started to use skimmed milk and substitute fruit with dry cereal for one egg about twice a week.
>
> He is not even an ounce overweight but the amount of high cholesterol foods in his diet worries me. I even suggested that he make a night appointment to donate a pint of blood, and get the laboratory to test his cholesterol. He refuses. I would blame myself partially if I were to allow him to continue eating these foods that might cause a heart attack.

I replied as follows:

> I commend you for your normal apprehension, but I am afraid that you may already be suffering from cho-

lesterolophobia. These days many a man is conscience-stricken when he butters his toast, orders eggs and bacon for breakfast, eats ice cream. He has been reading about the connection of saturated fats (such as these) and heart attacks.

Framingham (Massachusetts) and other studies certainly label fats as being potentially guilty. But I think too many are unnaturally fearful. Your husband, as you suggest, should have a periodic physical examination and a thorough cholesterol reading. But if it and the rest of the examination are normal, then let him enjoy his food—as he seems to be doing. However, if the doctor finds definite contraindications to his present high-fat intake, I would be the first to agree that he had better follow a low-fat, low-cholesterol diet.

But enough of cholesterolophobia; what about pain in the chest? It is the most common immediate cause of imaginary heart trouble. It brings more frightened patients to the doctor than any other symptom. Any discomfort in the left side of the chest is suspect. Each worried patient describes his symptoms in his own fashion: "It stabs me like a knife . , ." "It's a dull ache all day long . . ." "It's like painful collection of gas under my heart."

In my experience a safe guess is that eighty percent of such patients with "pain on the left side" do not have organic heart disease. A complete workup usually proves the hunch is correct.

I believe that thousands of doctors could cure hundreds of thousands of imaginary heart trouble patients tomorrow if it were possible to convince laymen to forget the difference between *left* and *right*.

For patients quickly overlook pain on the right side of the chest. A man will say he sprained a right-sided muscle while playing tennis or pushing a stalled car. But if his *left* chest hurts he forgets tennis and the car and fixes his mind on his heart.

Once I treated a patient who was certain that the fleeting pains in his left chest were due to heart disease. But he recovered quickly when he learned that he was one of the unusual people who had dextrocardia (a right-sided heart).

"That convinces me," he said. "Now I know it can't be my heart."

It is well to remember that organic heart pains usually fit into a definite diagnostic pattern. For instance, the pains of angina pectoris, coronary occlusion, aneurysm, or valvular disease are readily recognized by the competent physician. But when the patient takes upon himself the awesome responsibility to differentiate the real from the imaginary, unnecessary confusion and apprehension result.

Pain due to real heart disease usually is an unmistakable symptom. For instance, in coronary occlusion (sometimes called thrombosis or infarction) the discomfort usually spreads over the entire chest. It may last for hours with deepening intensity, broken by short intervals of freedom from extreme pain. In the patient with angina pectoris the periodic chest pains that follow exertion and excitement are also like carbon-paper replicas of preceding attacks under similar conditions.

But you should remember that, except for these coronary pains and occasional heart-valve disease pains, heart disease does not cause pain. The most common culprit is the mind which translates every chest discomfort into actual heart disease.

Do you recall the "stitch in your side" which you often got as a child? And how you forgot about it when the

80

pain passed? Somehow, too many of us grownups persist in associating similar innocuous chest pains with real heart disease. Doctors themselves may not be free from such fears.

I recall as vividly as if it were yesterday a doctor who sat across from my desk about twenty-five years ago. Outwardly, he had always appeared to be a carefree, fun-loving fellow. He would be the last you would expect to fall prey to anxiety. Yet, there he was, fidgeting in a chair, swabbing with his handkerchief at the sweat pouring down his face, his hand visibly shaking, and his voice so hushed and fearful I had to bend over to hear him.

"You don't know how much I appreciate your seeing me on such short notice," he said. "But I just had to come right away. Believe it or not, I'm afraid of dropping in my tracks. I never felt this way before. I was up until midnight with a very sick patient. Then I was called out twice on night emergencies, so I have had very little sleep."

He paused a second or two to marshal his thoughts, licking his lips nervously, then continued: "When I got out of bed this morning, I suddenly felt a twinge of pain in my left side. It was like a blunt scissors being stuck into me and separated in my chest. I sat there on the edge of the bed practically unable to breathe. My heart started pounding and the pricks of pain kept coming on. My wife was making breakfast. I did not call down to disturb her. I went to the bathroom and my reflection in the glass frightened me. I was pale, sweating, and as scared as any patient I have ever seen in my own practice.

"I took a hot shower, let the hot steam converge on my chest. When I got out to rub down, most of the pain had disappeared. But it didn't go away entirely. Since I am only thirty-eight, have a fine family and a lot to live for, I've kept worrying that I might be experiencing some kind of heart attack. That's why I've bothered you on such short notice."

And he looked at me imploringly, as I've seen so many frightened laymen look. His round, cherubic face had none of the usual laugh wrinkles I had seen whenever I passed him in a hospital corridor or at medical meetings.

I learned that he hadn't taken a vacation in a half-dozen years. He worked, as the saying goes, day and night as a busy general practitioner. He admitted to having felt exhausted for the past few weeks.

I looked him over carefully. There was no evidence of heart disease or of any other ailment. Nevertheless, I put him through a series of careful tests. An hour later, when I had finished, we went back to my consultation room and sat down.

I offered him a cigarette and lit my own (a quarter of a century ago few if any doctors associated cigarette-smoking with lung cancer, emphysema, or heart disease). I knew how a judge must feel before handing down a decision to the prisoner standing in the dock. His eyes burned into mine, as if this was the only support he had which prevented him from toppling out of his chair.

Therefore, I came right out with my decision: "Absolutely no evidence of heart disease." He almost collapsed, even on hearing good news. As doctor to doctor, I reviewed the results of every test I had made. Above all, I kept repeating that he must know, as a doctor, that the modern physician doesn't prevaricate when he has discovered heart disease in his patient. He comes right out with the truth,

"You don't have heart disease. If you did, I'd tell you. Stabs in the chest like yours come and go, and most of the time, we don't know the reason. But that's unimportant.

What IS important is that you wipe heart disease out of your mind.

"And I'll tell you how to begin. Make plans to get away for at least two weeks for that long-needed vacation. Not because you need a rest for heart *disease*—but because you need a rest for heart *trouble*. It's in your mind. And your mind is one big residue of fatigue. You're so exhausted that any other symptoms might throw you into some kind of panic.

"If you had belched a few times this morning you might have been sure you had gallstones. If you had had a twinge of pain in your stomach, you would have been fearful of having an ulcer.

"So, I repeat, take a holiday. You will not be able to run away from yourself, but you will find yourself as healthy as you used to be, after you refill your energy bank again."

Within days, he and his wife and two children went off on a two-week cruise. When he returned I was the first one he called.

"You've lost a patient," he said, a high ebullience in his voice. "But you've converted a damn fool into some kind of more sensible guy. From now on I'm going to respect just how much of a beating my body and mind can take. I've lost all fear of my heart. It has all been in my tired mind. From now on I'll be taking at least one long yearly vacation and some long weekends, too. Meanwhile, thanks for putting some sense into me."

Sometimes chest pain is so extreme and debilitating that it closely resembles an attack of coronary thrombosis. Neither the patient nor his doctor can be blamed for believing the trouble is heart disease and not due to trouble outside the heart.

One afternoon my wife received a long-distance call

from a close friend who was greatly disturbed because her husband had suffered a sudden pain in the chest. It had been so bad he had moved over to her seat and she had driven him to the nearest hospital. When they arrived, attendants from the emergency room had had to carry him inside on a stretcher.

As my wife's friend described the scene after I took over the phone, the husband writhed in pain, sweated like a man caught in midday during a hot spell, and seemed critical enough to be placed under an oxygen tent.

Doctors came in and made a provisional diagnosis of heart attack probably due to the closing off of a coronary artery. They kept him quiet in bed. But reports of repeated electrocardiograms and blood specimens for enzyme reactions kept coming back negative. Even after two weeks, all tests were negative. They took a gall bladder X ray. This, too, was negative.

My wife's friend said they were going to do a gastro-intestinal X-ray series in a few days. She asked me what I thought of the idea, and I told her I concurred.

When they returned home, she showed me the X-ray report. They had found a large hiatal hernia. The man's stomach was way up in his chest. And they had attributed his "heart attack" to this sudden pressure in his chest by the overwhelming encroachment of stomach on heart and lungs in the chest cavity.

In his case, operation on the enlarged opening in the diaphragm seemed like excellent judgment. He recovered nicely and lived to a nice old age without having another episode of chest pain.

(Another graphic example of how a "sure" attack of coronary thrombosis was due to trouble elsewhere.)

Of course, not all patients with hiatal hernia have se-

84

vere chest pain. Some people are born with the abnormally large opening in the diaphragm where the esophagus passes through, and never realize they have it because they suffer no symptoms. It is discovered on routine X-ray investigation. Such people need not be concerned, nor do they need any treatment.

In others with moderately large openings, symptoms may arise because the opening is large enough to allow some part of the stomach or its omental apron to slip up into the chest cavity. This may interfere with normal digestion, often causing heartburn, gas, belching—but rarely acute, diffuse chest pain. Symptoms are worse at night, especially after a heavy meal, and when the patient lies flat in bed. Such patients usually find relief with simple medical treatment—taking small, frequent meals rather than one or two large ones. They are helped by sleeping high on two or three pillows to prevent slippage of a portion of the stomach into the chest, by taking antacids and antispasmodics, and by deleting such gas-producing foods as cabbage, beans, and radishes from their diet.

Some impatient persons are anxious to undergo surgery as soon as hiatal hernia is diagnosed. I do not advise this unless the surgeon finds a specific reason for operation, for example, such as my wife's friend had in suddenly being prostrated by chest pain due to a very large diaphragmatic hernia.

There are no oracles in medicine. The fact that a doctor is a professor, has treated royalty, or numbers the great and near-great among his patients does not guarantee that he exceeds in wisdom or medical experience hundreds of other doctors practicing in his special field.

No matter how renowned, a physician must have real humility and a realization of his shortcomings. Personally,

I like and respect the physician who uses such words as "if"—"it depends"—"nobody can be sure"—when he discusses illness.

Conversely, I distrust the doctor who knows it all, who never qualifies his diagnosis or treatment, who is opinionated and arrogant. As I mentioned earlier, you will be safer in the hands of the one who always questions his diagnosis and treatment until he can be completely certain about the accuracy of the first and the effectiveness of the second.

I recall the story of an eighty-two-year-old man who suddenly collapsed with severe chest pain while working in his little grocery store. The family doctor, a young, bright diagnostician, said the pain was due to a collapse of the lung. A professor in consultation from a neighboring university disagreed. He thought it a typical case of coronary thrombosis. Not until repeated electrocardiograms taken over a period of ten days proved negative did they think it safe to move the patient for chest X rays. These confirmed the young doctor's diagnosis.

The older doctor quickly admitted to the family that his own diagnosis was wrong. He was so impressed by the younger colleague's diagnosis and behavior that he invited him a few years later to become his associate in private practice.

Although lung collapse is a very uncommon condition, it is another potential suspect where pain occurs in the chest. Incidentally, this patient recovered nicely and lived one week short of his ninetieth birthday.

Recently I was asked if it is possible to live with a bullet in the heart. The man, a casual acquaintance, said, "I've made a bet with a friend. It's just for a dunkin' doughnut and a cup of coffee, so your decision won't really hurt either of us. He says it's possible to live with a bullet in the heart and I say it's preposterous. Who buys the coffee and doughnuts?"

Undoubtedly, it was his turn to pick up the check for the doughnuts and coffee. In the *Review of Modern Medicine* there appeared an abstract of a medical report from the *New England Journal of Medicine*. It was called "Missiles in the Heart," and was written by Edward F. Bland, M.D., and Gilbert W. Beebe, Ph.D.

The conclusion states that a foreign object in the heart apparently can be retained with little risk of disability. Large missiles should be removed and the patient assured that his heart's function will be normal. But smaller objects should be left alone.

Forty veterans of World War II with heart-imbedded missiles were studied. Removal of the missiles was successful in three of eight of the patients and abandoned in five.

The routine followed by the remaining veterans was normal except for the psychological strain of living with a bullet in the heart. A few had no complaints, but almost all of them experienced apprehension, low tolerance for work, and chest pain. Thirty of the men are fully employed, but five are totally disabled by an anxiety neurosis related to living with a bullet inside their hearts.

Studies reveal that none have heart enlargement, nor is there any evidence that the missile has migrated or caused infection or erosion in the heart.

As I look at the article, I see an X-ray picture of one of the men. It shows the shadow of the bullet in the wall of the heart muscle twenty years after the man was shot.

For those who are unnaturally apprehensive about their heart, there is a lesson in this report. It proves that the healthy heart will go on beating, missile imbedded in it or not. In these veterans, at least, it was the mind rather than the heart that needed help over these many years.

Although I think my readers will agree that their anxiety is a natural reaction to such an injury and the knowledge that "the bullet is still in there," what is also evident is that some take it in stride and others keep on worrying.

People often ask me why I make the distinction between fear and anxiety. "Aren't they both the same?" they ask.

I tell them it is all a matter of degree.

When you are walking through the bush and are confronted by a tiger ready to spring, that is FEAR—with four capital letters. But if you walk through the countryside, knowing that there is a man-eating tiger at large, you walk in anxiety. You remain anxious until the tiger is caught, or until you can get miles away from the danger area.

It's fear when you are confronted with a peril you can recognize (seeing the tiger ready to jump). But it's anxiety when you recognize the possibility of danger but don't know when it will come—or don't even know what the danger is. Psychologists call this "free-floating" anxiety.

Many of us worry ourselves sick because of anxiety produced by chest pains. We are scared and we do not know why. Either we haven't gone to the doctor for a diagnosis or, having received a favorable report, we still stay scared.

You would think a learned judge would have more sense, but anxiety invades any barrier. He was a bluff, hearty man, broad-shouldered, opinionated, and with a reputation for being self-assured and even-tempered. But as he faced me across the desk in my consultation room, he seemed oddly ill at ease and apprehension darkened his eyes. When he spoke he sounded apologetic.

"I've been having pains on and off. Little stabs over my left chest. They don't last long, but they have been annoying. At a gathering the other night, a friend who studies palmistry read my palm and told me my lifeline is very short. Since I'm only forty-three, I am quite interested. I know everyone has a different fingerprint; then why should God go to the trouble to keep our identity separate and not give us further information like lifelines to guide our lives? I hope you don't think I'm a kook, but you have had the opportunity to see people both coming into and leaving this world. What do you think of lifelines? Am I ready for a trip to a psychiatrist?"

Here we have an example of anxiety rather than fear. The judge continued to have a low opinion of his heart for a few months longer. Coming in every week or two just to talk and "ventilate" his family problems soon converted him from being a cardiophobe into a much happier individual. Like so many others, his "heart pains" originated elsewhere.

Dr. Harold M. Marvin, in his book *You and Your Heart,* put it this way:

> Usually a heart that seems to its owner to be in trouble isn't. This seeming paradox is explained by the fact that many of the irregularities of beat and rhythm to which the heart is subject occur in the absence of organic disease, while pain or discomfort often thought by laymen to be caused by a misbehaving heart are much more likely to originate in some other organs. All these things happen to perfectly healthy hearts, perhaps even more often than to hearts that are really in trouble.

In my experience the most frequent disease outside the heart that so often causes chest pain and simulates real heart is trouble in the gall bladder.

The differential diagnosis between coronary pain and gall bladder can often disturb the most brilliant diagnostician. We try not to forget the gall bladder as the culprit whenever chest pain is the presenting symptom. (I'll discuss this in a following chapter.)

However, there are other reasons for "painful chests" that simulate real heart disease. I'll show you how anxiety can build the blocks of concern in one patient, while similar symptoms in another are passed by as being relatively unimportant.

During one morning in my office I saw two patients with painful shoulder bursitis with referred discomfort in the chest. The first patient was a large, rotund engineer who had taken on the job of repainting and repapering his home.

"I wanted to do it for exercise," he said, "but it left me pretty sore all over with the reaching for the ceiling and the walls. One day, about a week later, I began to have this pain in my left shoulder. It went all the way into my chest. I took a half-dozen aspirin tablets a day, applied a heat pad, but nothing seemed to help. It got worse. So bad, in fact, that I can hardly move my left arm because of the pain.

"Now that almost two months have gone by without any improvement, I think it's about time I gave a doctor a chance to work some magic. The chest pain is there night and day. I know you'll take electrocardiograms and X rays, but I really think they'll be a waste of time. I'm sure in my own mind that I've developed coronary pain. Otherwise, why should it be so persistent?"

As he sat there, apparently making light of his condition, I could sense that he was a frightened man. His wife said that he had taken an extended leave of absence from his office because of the fear that he might suddenly keel over during an attack.

His history and findings were typical of an angry shoulder bursa. The bursitis had limited his shoulder motion so much that he had developed what we call a "frozen shoulder." Electrocardiograms and other examinations subsequently eliminated coronary disease as a cause of his painful shoulder and chest.

After months of physiotherapy and the use of corticosteroids, we finally thawed out the frozen joint. His pains disappeared. Not until then was he completely convinced that his heart disease was really bursitis.

The second patient was a thin, nervous, birdlike little man whom you might surely think would be the one to suffer from anxiety about his heart. He, too, had shoulder pain and chest pain. Not once did he mention any concern about his heart nor reveal any hidden anxiety about it.

The reason was evident. He had right-shoulder bursitis and not left-shoulder bursitis.

He said, "I've come in for some cortisone which I know is supposed to be good for bursitis. I've had it for about a week and want to catch it in time. The chest pain doesn't bother me. I know it can't be my heart because the painful shoulder is on my right side and not on the heart side." (If left-shoulder bursitis had been causing his symptoms, he probably would have worried about his heart interminably.)

I recall a fifty-year-old school teacher who had a habit of raising her eyebrows as she spoke. She had a constant look of surprise on her features. One day she came into my office, saying, "Well, I guess time has caught up with me. I'm in my menopause and, for the past few days,

I've had a distressing pain in my left chest. It keeps me from working and sleeping. It burns and aches. I've known for some time that coronary attacks are quite infrequent in younger women; but when we get older, we are likely to have as many attacks as men do. Frankly, I'm quite perturbed about it. Shall I give up my teaching job?"

In her case, the examination was completely negative except for an area of tenderness around her left chest. Although I gave her a heart-not-guilty-verdict, she left the office questioning my diagnosis. Three days later she returned. Now the burning in the chest was worse than the pain.

"I'm all broken out on this side," she said. "I wonder if this is shingles [herpes zoster]. I had an aunt who had it and it resembled this eruption."

I examined her, found the telltale rash of inflammatory blebs and scabs. This virus infection that follows the nerve pathways can cause severe pain, and one can readily understand a patient's concern when the pain is in the left chest (supposedly "over the heart").

In spite of the fact that her discomfort continued for several months, as it often does in elderly patients who develop herpes zoster, she was free from any concern about her heart thereafter. If her shingles had not been confined to her left side, I wonder if we might not have added another cardiophobe to our long list of sufferers.

Some persons associate any numbness or pain in the left arm with heart disease. They think they may be suffering from an attack of angina pectoris. I have observed such fears in people who had abnormal muscle pressure on the arm nerves—either in the shoulder region (scalenus anticus syndrome) or in the wrist (carpal tunnel syndrome). Whenever there is such trouble, the patient should consult with an orthopedist before accepting his anxieties about a failing heart. In many such patients, an operation to relieve nerve pressure has cleared up the symptoms and removed the anxiety about heart disease.

In the middle-aged and elderly, especially, there is another common reason for chest pain completely unassociated with heart disease. I refer to the hundreds of thousands of people who have spinal arthritis.

It is easily conceivable that the rough spurs and the deterioration of the bony support in the spine—so intimately connected with the nerves that leave the spinal column—may impinge on the nerves supplying the chest wall and may cause all manner of painful symptoms. "I must have heart disease," is the usual lament.

Show some of these patients X rays of the spine, with definite evidence of arthritic changes, and they lose all fear of heart disease as a cause of the chest discomforts. But others are not so easily convinced. They will rationalize in spite of negative findings on heart study.

"Of course, it's possible that my arthritis is causing the chest pains. But why are they mostly on the left side? Isn't it possible that I may have heart disease also?"

Of course it is possible. Since arthritis is so common in the elderly, it is not unlikely that they may have heart disease also. But negative findings on complete examination should banish such fears,

People with arthritis and chest pain, without heart disease, will never tell you that the chest pain is not worse on exertion. They will say that the pain is often influenced by change of position (which may be due to temporary relief of nerve pressure). They will say that aspirin often works like magic on their chest pains. They have no symptoms such as difficulty in walking, shortness of breath, cough, swelling of the ankles, or any other of the common complaints of actual heart-disease patients.

93

If you continue to have anxiety about your heart even though your doctor has tried to reassure you that it is in excellent working order, I hope you will reread this chapter. The case histories I have presented have come from my files and from letters received from readers all over the United States and Canada. Compare your symptoms with theirs.

Perhaps you will accept the truth that chest pain is not invariably due to a weak heart. It should give you confidence to realize that hundreds of thousands of others who have also worried about their hearts have at last been convinced that this wonderfully strong muscular pump was still performing its incredible job.

6.

IT'S NOT ALWAYS AS
"EASY AS BREATHING"

Some patients call it the "shakes." Others say "I've got the jitters." Whatever the manifestations of discomfort, if the doctor looks and listens carefully, he often discovers that the patient is physically well but emotionally ill. And such illness varies in intensity.

All emotionally disturbed patients are not candidates for imaginary heart trouble. You can be normally disturbed: for example, scared of the "bomb" and its potentialities for destruction. In fact, I believe that much of modern tension derives from this unconscious fear which we all have. Fortunately, most of us handle it better than those who live in daily anxiety.

Has your machine been sputtering lately? Are you unduly concerned that something beyond repair is endangering your heart and your life? Don't despair. Millions in the United States like you have become alarmed by trifling symptoms. Not trifling in the sense that they *imagine* the discomforts—but trifling in a medical sense. We physicians know you may have such symptoms and still be basically healthy.

A common complaint of anxious people is that they

can't breathe. And knowing that shortness of breath is a common symptom of heart disease, they bear the burden of this diagnosis even before they have consulted a physician.

I recall so many anxious persons who said, "I can't breathe. I can't seem to take a full breath and really fill my lungs with air." Others would say, "I can't breathe. I'm short of breath." As if to prove it, they would sit there sighing deeply and visibly struggling to take a deep breath. Then they would throw their hands up in defeat, shrug their shoulders as if to say, "See? I told you I can't do it."

These are not evidences of shortness of breath due to physical illness. They are surface indications of submerged anxiety. They are proof that "it's easy as breathing" is a misnomer. When emotions go berserk, breathing may go berserk. Sometimes we do not realize that either our emotions or breathing is out of order until it is pointed out to us by the doctor.

An important example of this is the syndrome doctors call "hyperventilation." Here is such a patient:

She sits in my consultation room on the edge of her chair. She is tense and her features are rigid with fear. She is in her mid-thirties, pretty, well dressed, and quite able to communicate.

"I suppose you are tired, doctor, of trying to help us frightened individuals. You have so little time and need it for those more seriously ill. Nevertheless, I am selfish enough to demand your precious time because I feel much sicker than I may appear to be. As a wife of a fine husband and three children, I owe it to them—if not to myself—to be freed from my fears.

"During the past six months I do not recall one day

96

that I have felt calm and relaxed like most normal persons do. What I wouldn't give to be like that again. [Now that she had begun to talk, she became less rigid, slipped back into the chair, and talked less rapidly.]

"My trouble is simply fear. I live scared. I'm convinced that my heart may give out momentarily. For this reason I've had to give up so much of my social life. I never go out to play golf because I'm afraid I'll collapse on a fairway, far from the aid of a doctor.

"When I have been sufficiently coaxed to go to the movies or the theater, I insist on sitting close to the back row and in an aisle seat, so I can rush outside when the fear suddenly envelops me.

"When panic strikes me, my heart begins to race and pound. I feel faint and have to actually hold onto an imaginary object to brace myself against falling to the floor. I break out into a sweat. My hands and feet tingle and feel numb.

"I know what you will say. You'll probably repeat what other doctors have already told me. They say that my heart's all right and it's only my nerves. Tranquilizers haven't really helped. My children and husband still bear with me, but I know I'm not being fair to them by acting like this. I come to you as just another doctor in the long line I have already visited. What will the verdict be? Just nerves, again?"

I recall this patient vividly as she sat there, looking at me, waiting for any evidence that I might be prevaricating or passing out to her the usual "pap" such patients often receive: "You'll be all right. Just stop worrying."

"I've listened to your story patiently," I said. "I hope you'll listen to what I have to say. As you have been talking, I've been observing you carefully. And I believe I have found two important clues that may help solve this mystery of yours.

"First, I notice that you sigh a lot. You've punctuated practically every other sentence by a long, deep sigh—of which you are probably unaware. Second, between sighs, I note that you take fast, shallow breaths. Instead of the normal number of respirations, you take at least thirty-five to forty breaths a minute.

"Now, you may wonder what all this has to do with your fears for your heart and your life. If what my hunch says is true, then you have what we call hyperventilation —a common counterpart of the anxiety state from which patients like yourself suffer."

She gazed at me with an expression one sees in a child who has been given an explanation which is above and beyond her comprehension. Nevertheless, she remained quiet.

"I'll try to give you some definite proof that what I say is not something far out. With your cooperation I'll conduct an experiment, here and now, to convince you that your anxiety about your heart is due to hyperventilation. Later on, I'll explain just what hyperventilation is all about. But now for the experiment."

I asked her to take forcibly deep breaths, in and out, in and out—as many as she could per minute—for at least two or three minutes. I promised that she would soon experience exactly the same symptoms that she complained of in the theater, in a crowd—or anywhere. I told her she would suddenly begin to feel faint, perspire, have palpitation and all the rest of the fearsome symptoms that she usually had with these attacks.

She complied. She cooperated beautifully. Within two minutes she clutched at her left chest, reached her right hand out to the desk for support and said, "Doctor, do something. I'm going. I'm going." Her pulse was at least 180 and she had stiffened in fright.

I had a brown, paper bag ready, told her to breathe and rebreathe into it for a few minutes, and the attack of panic was soon over.

We sat looking at one another. She soon responded to my smile of encouragement and said, "It's almost unbelievable. I mean producing, so dramatically and truly, the symptoms I've been complaining about. And ending the attack so quickly by breathing into an ordinary supermarket bag. It's fantastic."

I told her it was now time for an explanation of hyperventilation itself. Unless she knew the physiological implications of overbreathing, the hyperventilation would still be a mystery and she would not benefit from the experiment we had just performed.

I said, "Hundreds of thousands of anxiety-burdened persons suffer from hyperventilation unknowingly. Often, until lately, it has been overlooked by physicians themselves. Patients with this condition often suffer from chronic fear of heart disease because their pulse races, they feel faint, complain of chest pain and fatigue, and perspire unduly. These people unconsciously overbreathe—too fast and too often. Sometimes, deeply and slowly, by sighing frequently. Or by yawning often.

"What is the actual result of all this unnatural intake and expulsion of air? We call it an oxygen-carbon dioxide imbalance. Too much carbon dioxide is forced out of the body by rapid breathing. As a result, the carbon dioxide tensions in the small lung cells called the alveoli, and in the blood, become much lower than normal. What follows is a lessened supply of needed oxygenated blood to the tissues, especially to the brain. This brings about the symptoms patients complain about."

I went on: "It is true that most people do recover from an acute anxiety attack without breathing and rebreathing into a paper bag. But this simple technique works so quickly to eliminate anxiety symptoms because it restores the oxygen–carbon dioxide balance in the blood by offering a reserve amount of carbon dioxide which the blood has lost. As a result, the brain gets its quota of necessary oxygen and behaves accordingly."

I concluded our meeting by impressing upon her the importance of becoming aware of how she breathed. She was one of the fortunate ones who was able, within a few weeks, to retrain her breathing habits. She would know immediately if she was breathing too often. She learned to use diaphragmatic breathing rather than shallow chest breathing.

Soon her symptoms had evaporated and disappeared. No longer did she have any fears of being in public—or by herself. Panic no longer overwhelmed her. Although still occasionally anxious, she no longer had a loss of confidence in the performance and strength of her heart.

Not all patients improve so dramatically and so quickly. Hyperventilation itself may, in some individuals, be a part of a deep-seated emotional disturbance. Relieving the hyperventilation does help, but only partially. The job remains for the physician to treat the whole patient for any residual weaknesses in the patient's personality.

If you have been overbreathing it is important for your doctor to determine what psychological problem you are attempting consciously or unconsciously to overcome. He must try to discover what there is in your past, present, or fears for the future, which sets off the periodic explosions of overbreathing.

The doctor must dig deeply to find the cure. Remember that the hyperventilation syndrome may be but one part

100

of an anxiety reaction. I tell you this so you will be patient if the cure of hyperventilation doesn't immediately erase all symptoms.

The former case history illustrates that the art of medicine is really a mixture of the art and science of medicine. The doctor still needs to be aware of the human needs of his patient: He must understand his emotional problems, his fears and anxieties; and he must constantly bear in mind that he is treating a human being and not a guinea pig.

I have seen and known many patients who have improved (or completely recovered) after they became aware that hyperventilation was tied in with their anxiety. Most of all they asked, "Will I ever get over it? Or must I live and die with it?"

Here it is important to emphasize once again that the patient who has faith in his recovery has a much better likelihood of getting well than the pessimist and doubter. This is true of any kind of illness. My surgeon friends tell me that faith is similarly effective in surgical operations. They cross their fingers when a patient to be operated on says, "I don't think I'll ever come out of the anesthetic." The truth is that quite often it is this type of patient who gets complications and is a cause for worry.

Whatever your discomforts and your fears about your heart's capacity to carry on, you will overcome them more quickly if you face up to yourself and agree that "psychosomatics" is not just a fancy word dreamed up by the medical profession. It is based on experience and experiment.

I came across an interesting observation by a layman in a newspaper column recently: "I scarcely know a man past his middle thirties who has not had some lower back trouble; and most of them are suffering from little more than tension and anxiety. The common cause of 'illness' in this country lies in the head, not in the rest of the body."

Perhaps you will accept this truth coming from a layman more readily than when it comes from a doctor. Most people get their backs up when they are confronted with the word "psychosomatic" as characterizing the reason for faulty breathing and other heart symptoms.

Though I respect the next fellow's opinion, this doesn't mean that I invariably subscribe to it—whether he be layman or doctor. Recently I have been hearing and reading that some doctors believe the dangers of obesity have been overstressed. They say it is "natural" for some people to be fat. "Don't tamper with them. Let them eat in peace and grow fat."

Fortunately, this opinion is shared by only a minority of medical opinion. My own experience in practice—and borne out by insurance statistics and other data—has convinced me that if you allow yourself to get fat, you may invite trouble.

For example, I quote Dr. Stephen Smith of New York who, at the age of ninety-nine, said, "We should be in our prime at fifty and not begin to age until past eighty. Men who die at the usual age do so by their own knives and forks."

It is true that excess fat predisposes to atherosclerosis, coronary disease, stroke, gall bladder trouble, arthritis, diabetes, liver disease—you name it. The trouble with obesity is that so many do not consider it a dangerous disease in itself because it comes so stealthily, without pain. It is a friendly sort of enemy.

But, benign or not, obesity can be a threat to your peace of heart. I recall a rotund businessman who came in one day certain that he had developed heart disease.

"Shortness of breath is one of the main symptoms, isn't it?" he inquired.

I asked him when he noticed this symptom.

"Yesterday, for the first time," he replied, his rotund face showing concern. "As you know, we've had a strike of elevator operators, and I had to walk up six floors to my office. By the time I got to the third landing I was panting like a dog. When I reached the sixth floor, I almost collapsed. If that isn't an indication of heart trouble, I'd like to know what is."

All tests were negative. I told him that obese people, unused to exercise, often suffer shortness of breath after unusual physical activity. But he would not accept this explanation. In his mind, his shortness of breath that day was due to some sort of heart failure. Not until he took off about forty pounds during the next half-year was he convinced that his heart was all right. One day he made a trial rerun of his office stairs on my recommendation. He was able to skip up the six flights without resting, and as he said, "When I got up there I was ready for six more."

I tell other obese patients who base their anxiety on shortness of breath as an indication of heart disease, to reduce. This will convince them of their heart's capability more than negative reports on electrocardiograms and X rays. They will agree that excess poundage and loss of muscle tone are reason enough for their shortness of breath.

One way to prevent shortness of breath, then, is to stay near your normal weight. As one patient put it, "I've learned that it's easier not to start a bad habit like overeating than to stop it or cut down."

Samuel Johnson fathered a truism, a long medical sermon in a few words, when he said, "Abstinence is easier for me than temperance."

Anyone who has ever tried to smoke less will attest to the truth of this observation. Once the habit is formed and welded, it takes more than strength of will to become unshackled from it.

It is for this reason that I tell youngsters that it is easier not to begin to smoke than to moderate or stop after learning. And it is easier not to follow the crowd by taking those first few beers while in high school or college. Those first few drinks are fertile ground for the birth and growth of chronic alcoholism later. What goes for tobacco and alcohol is, of course, even more true for the habitual use of drugs.

And so it is with overweight. Begin to abstain from the excess calories long before the excess fat has spread in layers and has become a major reducing problem. Only in this way will you eliminate one of the symptoms that make for anxiety about heart function: shortness of breath.

Of course, most people attribute shortness of breath to obvious causes. They do not pin the label "heart disease" on themselves.

The fat man says, "I guess I'm too heavy to get around like I used to without getting short of breath." The middle-aged athlete who gets winded on the tennis court says, "I guess the ol' man isn't what he used to be."

Unfortunately, the chronically anxious will not accept such evident causes for their dyspnea.

Most asthmatic sufferers will say, "What bothers me most is my shortness of breath. I guess my lungs have gone back on me." Nevertheless, some asthmatics will immediately be suspicious that the trouble is in their heart and not so much in their lungs.

Take the following case involving a completely frustrated woman. She dabs at her eyes with her handkerchief as she tells me of her sixty-eight-year-old husband who suffers from emphysema and fullness in the chest. He is hardly able to work at his bakery trade, gets winded easily, coughs, and takes long breaths.

He has been this way, and getting worse, for five years. It takes him an hour or two in a warm room to get his breath. Sometimes he can hardly walk or talk. He goes to a clinic only once a year for a checkup although they want to see him at least every two weeks. He probably stays away so he won't hear them say to stop smoking. He is a chain smoker, although he knows it's killing him.

I told her that I could not answer her question about how he got the emphysema. All we know is that it is four or five times more frequent in men than in women. Often the cause is obscure; however, most patients reveal a long history of smoking cigarettes, or having had bronchitis, asthma, or frequent attacks of pneumonia. The chronic cough aggravates the disease, and some medical people think actually causes it.

Another emphysema patient who came to my attention was wrong at first and right at last. A truck driver by trade, he was a three-pack-a-day smoker from his early twenties. By the time he was in his late forties he began to complain of severe breathing distress on exertion. "It must be my heart," he concluded.

Although he was told that he had an unmistakable case of emphysema, he continued to berate his heart as letting him down. Perhaps it was his way of rationalizing away cigarettes as the contributing cause of his shortness of breath.

"Why give up cigarettes when the trouble is in my heart and not in my lungs," he kept saying.

By the time he was fifty-two years of age, he was so

105

short of breath that he could not walk twenty-five yards without resting. Even when he was sitting quietly at home, without having made any recent exertions, you could see him fight to take in and expel air. His lips were blue, and as he breathed, his shoulders would move up and down in an effort to assist his overworked lungs.

Now, however, after having put extra pressure on his breathing apparatus for so many years, he was being proved correct. His heart was beginning to fail, too. He was having right-sided heart failure, which doctors call "cor pulmonale."

As one can readily see, untreated emphysema in a habitual heavy smoker invariably gets worse. Early diagnosis and treatment are essential. But like the alcoholic who wants to get better (and must first admit that he is an alcoholic) the emphysema patient with shortness of breath must be willing to admit that at first the trouble is in his lungs—long before he blames his innocent heart muscle for lack of tenacity and unwillingness to work.

The chief aim of the expert in chest diseases who treats the emphysema patient for shortness of breath is to try to prevent the complicating stages of the disease that are characterized by drowsiness, headache, cyanosis, and actual unconsciousness due to lack of oxygen and trapped carbon dioxide. These are the forerunners of distinct bronchial obstruction that cause the increase of carbon dioxide in the blood and the development of right heart failure.

As a rule, patients with emphysema become easily discouraged. I remind them that the illness has been years in developing; that they should not expect or hope that their breathing will become easier within weeks or a few months. Even their lack of appetite, loss of strength, and sleeplessness resist treatment at first.

106

But we do not give up in treating emphysema as easily as we did only a few years back. If your present doctor hasn't the capabilities or equipment for modern diagnosis and treatment you should consult a chest specialist. It is his job to determine how much functional capacity remains in your lungs.

He has the apparatus in his office to determine such complicated functions as vital capacity, tidal volume, inspiratory capacity, expiratory reserve volume—all important in assessing your lungs' ability to work. He may also do a bronchoscopic examination, take X rays and blood tests to round out the investigation.

Once he has diagnosed emphysema, you can bet your dollars to proverbial doughnuts that he will advise you to "stop all smoking" (most emphysema patients are habitual users of the weed). He may prescribe special medicines called aerosols (which are mist-carrying medications) that you can administer to yourself by hand bulb manipulation, to be inhaled during the day or night. These bring relief by dilating your bronchi and allowing them to bring more air to the lungs. Oxygen, special exercise, antibiotics, epinephrine, and other drugs are also used to help the breathing of the emphysema patient.

If your doctor says your breathing difficulty is due to trouble in your lungs, and not in your heart, better believe him. If you don't, you may be right, later on, when the weakness has extended to your heart.

Whatever interferes with normal breathing, day in and day out, may lay the basis of fear about the capacity of one's heart. In the person susceptible to anxiety, anything from unaccommodation to ordinary exercise all the way to the emphysema patient struggling for breath is sufficient to make him a cardiophobe who distrusts his own heart.

I tell such patients that they should not cling to guilt

feelings that they are unnecessary appendages of society. If they overcome their fears, they can still work and produce important projects—in spite of their apparent helplessness. Neither should they squirm in shame if someone calls them neurotics.

Marcel Proust has said, "Everything great in the world comes from neurotics. They alone have founded our religions and composed our masterpieces. Never will the world know all it owes them nor all they have suffered to enrich us. We enjoy lovely music, beautiful paintings, a thousand intellectual delicacies, but we have no idea of their cost, to those who invented them, in sleepless nights, tears, spasmodic laughter, rashes, asthmas, epilepsies, and the fear of death, which is worse than all the rest."

Proust speaks, of course, about the anxious human beings who have had the talent and the genius to make large contributions to the world. But think of the unknown and the unnamed whose fear of heart weakness and of death is so great that they consider it a great feat to have the courage to get out of bed in the morning and show up for work.

If you multiply or rearrange, as in a pack of cards, all the combinations of ways that anxiety slices off large chunks of satisfactory living from the lives of so many persons, you will realize that imaginary heart trouble (and other anxieties) anesthetizes the senses against enjoyment of living.

G. M. Beard, writing of psychoneuroses back in 1881, said, (calling it "American nervousness"):

> All this is modern and originally American; and no age, no country, and no form of civilization, not Greece, nor Rome, nor Spain, nor the Netherlands,

in the days of their glory, possessed such maladies. Of all the facts of modern sociology this rise and growth of functional nervous disease is one of the most stupendous, complex, and suggestive.

I doubt that the United States is the only country where people worry about themselves. But we certainly have our share of anxious people. Heart worriers certainly are legion. Faint-hearted people, because of their fears about their heart's function, will agree that half-living is half-dying.

They go through the motions but are like puppets on a string. They walk, they dance, they smile, they work, they play—but somehow they are empty of feeling. Ask the man who is about to walk the last mile how his dinner tastes. Ask the man who thinks his shortness of breath is sure augury of his last day on earth. How can he possibly enjoy himself—as he seems to be doing. As he himself will admit, "All I do is go through the motions of living."

Here is a letter I received some time ago from a visibly frightened woman:

> For the past seven or eight months I've not cared much about anything or anyone in my life. As a matter of fact, my very first words or thoughts upon awakening each morning are, "I wish I were dead."
>
> I mean it with all my heart. And speaking of my heart, I guess that's where it all started—one morning when I got short of breath carrying two heavy grocery bags into the house. I sat down, frightened that my heart was giving out, and I've been scared of my heart since.
>
> I've been to four doctors who have taken tests and examined me, and they all have come up with the same diagnosis, "You have a nervous heart."
>
> I'm a woman forty-six years of age, married to the

best husband in the world, with two grown daughters aged seventeen and nineteen. I know I'm going through my change but I also know that this is not my problem.

What bothers me is my heart. And the problem is compounded by something which may seem silly and unimportant to you. I've always been a very nervous and emotional person. (That's why I say it isn't the menopause that is bothering me.) As I said, what you may think is ridiculous is that I was a very attractive woman and I'm not any longer.

I understand we all get older and lose our looks and figures but in my case it happened overnight— on the day I suffered that shortness of breath attack. I fell aleep that night and woke up several hours later with a funny feeling around my lips. Sure enough, now my mouth seems to have that turned down ("sad clown") look ever since. It has made my whole face take on a crabby look at all times.

I'm ugly and can't take it. I know I'm not imagining it because I look in the mirror and mirrors don't lie! When I come home from shopping, I cry my heart out.

In spite of this woman's protestations that it "wasn't the menopause" she was really suffering from involutional melancholia (a rare complication of the menopause) as I later determined when she came to me for treatment. Her symptoms of depression intensified so much that I prescribed electric-sleep therapy. This treatment, combined with proper hormones and tranquilizing therapy, gradually restored her to her former "beauteous self" and removed all fears that her heart was malfunctioning.

I recall a young girl—slender and blonde with blue eyes and pale, smoothly textured skin—who nursed her ailing mother for months. She gave up college at the end

110

of her sophomore year, tended house, sat by her mother's beside for hours reading to her, while her mother sat up in bed, propped by several pillows, trying to catch her breath because of a failing rheumatic heart.

Because there were only the two of them, the responsibility (which she accepted readily and with love) fell on her alone. When she went to sleep at night the last thing she heard was her mother's labored breathing, and it was the first thing she heard on waking in the morning.

Is it any surprise, then, that she came to my office a few weeks after her mother's death, saying: "I'm so frightened I can't bear to go on living like this. My breathing bothers me. I can't catch a deep breath. It's like the trouble my mother had breathing before she died. I'm sure it must be my heart. I've been to one doctor who says it's due to nerves. I cannot understand how nerves can make a person feel the way I do constantly.

"From morning till night I feel groggy and dizzy. I am extremely despondent and have the urge to scream or run to get away from myself. I break out in cold sweats when I think of my heart. My legs get weak and I go completely numb. My throat feels tight, and my muscles ache as if I'm coming down with influenza at times.

"I feel like I'm alone in my problem; especially when the last doctor put the label on me: 'You're just a neurotic.' I know he did his best. He took two X rays and three electrocardiograms, but I'm not convinced that nerves can do all this. Why should I wake with palpitations and shortness of breath at night and fear that my heart will stop beating?" She stopped, breathless and despondent, her blue eyes now dark with pain and misery. Then she added in a low, broken voice, "It begins to look as if no one can help me."

Nevertheless, within three months this girl was back in

111

college and playing tennis, dancing, and entering class activities, her features and her entire manner reflecting her restored vigor and happy outlook on life. A magic cure? You might call it so, but the method was simple.

A combination of the doctor's "big ears" and a clear-cut demonstration that many of the symptoms were due to hyperventilation. As she talked her problem out with me, it at last became evident to her that one would have to be strong-willed, indeed, not to have "sympathetic symptoms" similar to those borne by a mother one had nursed for so many months.

Like Hippocrates, we have at last learned that doctors must treat the whole man—his mind as well as his body. As you can see, sometimes he even has to learn to breathe again before he loses his anxieties.

7.

DO YOU REALLY HAVE
A HEART COUGH?

Isn't it frustrating when you've had a toothache and it disappears completely by the time you sit down in your dentist's chair?

—When you have been having heart skips for a few days and you become frightened, you call your doctor's nurse and say, "I simply must have an appointment today. It's an emergency." You go to the doctor. He listens carefully, even takes an electrocardiogram—then no sign of a heart skip.

—When you are sure your eyesight is failing because you seem to need a stronger light to read by? You immediately think of glaucoma or a cataract. The doctor examines you. He says all you need is a change of lenses. Your vision is not greatly impaired.

—When you have been nagged by headaches day after day for at least two weeks. You sit in your doctor's waiting room thinking of high blood pressure, brain tumor, and all the rest. Your headache miraculously disappears. Your doctor says you never looked better in your life.

—When a persistent cough keeps you up nights. You

figure it might be due to too much smoking, but in the back of your mind is the frightening notion that it might signify lung cancer or heart disease. So you see your doctor and he tells you. "You're lucky everything is all right. But I'm not sure I can tell you the same unless you cut out your two-pack-a-day habit."

Don't feel foolish when symptoms disappear by the time you reach the doctor's office. Your doctor knows that nature plays tricks. Toothache, heart skips, vision, headache, coughs—all have a way of confusing you, but they don't throw your doctor off the diagnostic track. If there's one thing we learn by experience it is this: absence of symptoms and signs do not mean that a patient has been exaggerating or fabricating.

A toothache, headache, or cough is likely to return within minutes after the patient leaves the office. The heart skips may return the same night, while the patient is quietly resting in bed. So may the wracking cough. If there's a moral it is this: Don't hesitate to tell your doctor about your complaints even though they've disappeared temporarily.

But when you go in for a heart checkup because you are concerned that your cough may be due to a weak heart, and you are out of the doctor's office in 20 minutes, you haven't really had a careful survey. You have had only what some call a quick "look-see." The days are long gone when any medical practitioner, no matter how brilliant, can tap your chest a few times, lay on the stethoscope, and come up with a correct or reliable diagnosis of your heart's condition. History-taking requires, at the minimum, at least a half hour.

In addition, you should have a fluoroscopic examination, an X ray of the chest, electrocardiograms, and indicated laboratory tests. There may be special reasons later for

114

"barium swallows" while being fluoroscoped, for cardiac catheterization in suspected congenital heart patients, and for many other special investigative maneuvers.

A heart examination, to be worth anything, must be thorough. Don't go looking for "bargains" when the question of your heart's future is at stake.

Although a cough is not so common a symptom in heart disease as chest pain, shortness of breath, palpitation, it, nevertheless, frightens many susceptible people into believing that they do have heart disease.

I recall one such patient who wanted an examination but hesitated to submit to X rays of his chest. He was a dark-browed, heavy-chested insurance salesman in his mid-forties, with a thin gray moustache and a bright red tie, that seemed to be reflected from a large red nose.

During the consultation in my office he immediately voiced his fears. "I'm so afraid of X rays that I have even refused to let my dentist take a picture of a recalcitrant tooth that has been keeping me up nights. I know I'm being silly. I suppose I'll have to take your word for it that the X rays of my chest that you propose are necessary. I'll have them, but I'm still scared. It all started when a friend said that I've already had my safe quota of X rays this year. I had a GI series, a barium enema, and X rays for a twisted ankle. He said taking another X ray (even of a tooth) might get me into radiation difficulty."

I told him that many others like him wonder if they are getting a radiation overdosage. The decision should be left to a professional man rather than to a well-meaning friend. Until a few years ago old-fashioned X-ray machines were still around and were manned by people inexperienced in radiology. It is possible that a few patients received more exposure than was necessary.

115

But that is a rare probability today. All you need to do is seek out a reputable physician, one well trained in radiology, and you can put your confidence in him and in his equipment.

I sent out the man with the red nose and red tie to an X-ray specialist who found no evidence of trouble in the lungs or heart. Needless to say, the patient was thankful that he had the pictures and that they "turned out pretty."

In a recent *Bulletin of the American College of Radiology* there was this quotation from testimony before the United States Senate by Dr. Richard H. Chamberlain:

> "We think that the public has the right to expect protection against harmful amounts of inadvertent exposure to radiation from the operation of electronic devices. The risks to patients in the performance of medical X-ray examinations are vanishingly small. Diagnostic X-ray examinations do not endanger the health of patients, despite a few shrill claims to the contrary. We could cite millions of instances where X-ray examinations provide lifesaving information to patients."

It seems evident, then, that if you have any doubts about the cause of your cough, you should not allow any undue fears about X rays to influence your decision.

If you have a cough, consider it a friend rather than an enemy. It is a symptom or a warning, not trouble. It points the yellow arrow at something going on. However, if you have made your own diagnosis that your cough is due to a failing heart muscle, it's time that you realize a cough is present in many diseases and non-diseases. For example, a disease: lung cancer; a non-disease: tension.

First, what is a cough? It is sort of an explosion of air as a part of your respiratory system tries to rid itself of

116

some irritating material. It may be a crumb of bread that has "gone down the wrong way" or some mucus due to an infection.

You take a deep breath, and involuntarily close the top of the windpipe which we call the epiglottis; then you squeeze hard with the chest and belly muscles. The result is a sudden opening of the top of the windpipe and air is forced out at a speed of more than 250 miles an hour, expelling the irritating material (or at least attempting to do so). A cough may be loose or dry, depending upon its cause. If it lasts for more than a week or two, better have yourself checked. If you are fearful that it is a heart cough, all the more reason for not procrastinating.

Don't be one of the millions of Americans who spend about two billion dollars every year on self-prescribed cough mixtures. And don't buy cough medicine "just like the medicine" that helped your neighbor's cough. Some people do so to save money (but spend more on needless mixtures than they might by seeing a doctor in the first place). Others are too frightened to go because they can't face a possible serious diagnosis. I have known some who procrastinated simply because they were too ashamed to expose themselves during a physical examination. Prudery keeps some people from getting well.

I recently received a note from a woman that illustrates the fact that many patients are extremely uncomfortable during visits to their doctor:

> I have been bothered by a bad cough and some shortness of breath for a few weeks, and have been secretly thinking it's my heart.
>
> My own doctor referred me to a specialist. He is a fine man, yet I don't want to return to see him. During the examination, I am left completely exposed.

117

Since I have large, pendulous breasts, I am self conscious.

He doesn't put on a drape. His nurse, who is his wife, doesn't even come into the examining room. I am embarrassed. I should think he'd insist on covering me with a sheet. I'm sure it doesn't enter his mind that he is causing me this discomfort.

I've wanted to ask him to cover me, but I'm afraid he'd think I was suggesting something that isn't my business. Do you think I'd be wrong to make this suggestion? My family doctor always uses a sheet. His nurse is always in the room. I'd hate to have to give up the specialist now. My health is better, thanks to him. I cough less and fear for my heart less, because I believe in him. But how can I go about telling him without hurting his feelings?

In my reply I told her that if she likes the specialist she should speak out and tell him how she feels. He will appreciate it. But if there is something she does not like, such as not being covered by a sheet, being examined without the presence of a nurse, or being kept waiting for hours in his office—then she should not hesitate to make her feelings known to him.

She followed my advice and made a special friend out of the specialist, who appreciated her frankness. In fact, it caused him to change his office routine in the examination of patients. What was more important was his ability to convince her that her occasional spells of coughing were due to an allergy rather than to a weakening heart muscle.

I am not suggesting that any cough should be underrated. There must be a reason for the sale of an estimated six hundred varieties of cough mixtures over the counter without prescription. This is only catch-as-catch-can treatment that may temporarily disguise significant underlying trouble.

Anyone who coughs persistently is liable to have immediate complications such as insomnia, nausea, headaches, fainting spells, hemorrhage, hernia—even a fracture of a rib. But it is the long-term complications like heart disease (cor pulmonale) or emphysema (due to the stretching and breaking down of so many of the weakened, tissue-thin walls of the lungs' alveoli) against which precautions must be taken.

You need not go running to the doctor for every little cough. Nevertheless, early diagnosis is important—especially if you live in daily fear that the cough and any associated shortness of breath indicate heart disease.

I have indicated elsewhere that I try not to pat people on the back reassuringly at all times, as if to indicate that it isn't possible that their heart symptoms may not really be due to a failing heart. If I did so, my patients would not believe me even when I was telling them the truth.

Therefore, in discussing coughs it is not fair to keep giving examples of coughs "not due to heart disease" without including evidence that a cough can be a symptom of actual heart disease, too.

For example, I recall a nervous little man in his fifties, owner of a small hardware store, who complained of an irritating cough "that a dozen previous doctors couldn't cure." It persisted. It kept him up nights. He was getting desperate because of his insomnia and chronic fatigue.

He was especially despondent because he had quit his two-pack-a-day habit. "You would think," he said petulantly, "that with this sacrifice of my only remaining pleasure in life, the cough would go away."

But it clung stubbornly. In his mind it proved he didn't

119

have a "nervous" cough, as so many doctors had labeled it. Others said it was just a bad nervous habit. One said it was due to chronic bronchitis. Whatever the diagnostic tag, the cough held on. Cough mixtures and sedatives were of no avail.

By the time he came to see me, many months after having visited his twelfth doctor, much of the diagnostic ground had been furrowed. It was comparatively easy for me to try a new remedy. His previous blood tests, electrocardiograms were negative. X rays showed some fluid at the lung bases. Listening with the stethoscope I could easily hear some moist rales. Pressing with my thumb, there was unquestionable pitting edema of his ankles. The X rays also showed that there was some enlargement of the heart.

Had he been suffering from congestive failure of the heart all along? Was the cough a "heart cough"? I prescribed digitalis and diuretics (to remove excess fluid). Within a week, the cough that had been unremitting had completely disappeared.

Digitalis had exerted its effect on the heart to make it beat more strongly, to drive the excess fluid out of the lung sacs. And the diuretics completed the job. Once the irritating effects of excess, unnatural fluids had been removed, the cough was overcome as if a magic wand had caused it to vanish.

He said, "You're a miracle man."

I replied, "Any doctor who was doctor number thirteen could have helped as well."

When the heart is strong, you can run without getting too winded; you can eat heavily without suffering indigestion (unless there is another cause for indigestion); you can lie flat and still breathe easily; you can work hard without getting tired; you can stand and walk and run, yet your ankles will not swell. You will not develop a "heart cough."

But when the heart muscle begins to weaken, it cannot pump blood efficiently. Tissues do not get their full complement of oxygen. Important salts, minerals, chemicals, hormones, vitamins are not at the right place at the right time in the right quantities. In other words, circulation becomes disrupted, and this influences the state of the lungs, liver, and all other organs.

As a result, in congestive heart failure, fluid begins to collect at the bottom of the lungs, causing a chronic cough and shortness of breath, inability to lie flat and to perform any unusual exertions. The liver becomes congested and enlarged. So does the heart. The legs become edematous (filled with fluid—which usually disappears after leg elevation and a night's rest). The cough may be overlooked as being the result of a failing heart.

The doctor's most important job is to discover the cause of the heart failure. What kind is it? Hypertensive heart disease? Coronary artery disease? Rheumatic heart disease? Congenital heart disease? Bacterial endocarditis? Or isn't the cough due to heart disease at all?

Although prescribing digitalis and other drugs which strengthen the heart and help remove excess fluid is essential, what is as important is to treat the underlying cause of the heart disease: for example, antihypertensive drugs for high blood pressure, antibiotics for rheumatic heart disease. Remember that congestive heart failure is an all-inclusive term for weakness in many types of heart disease.

Many imaginary heart patients are nevertheless unaware that their cough is due to trouble in the lungs and not the result of some malfunction of the heart. And they are especially apt to overlook the possibility that they may be suffering from bronchial trouble.

Bronchitis is a label we often apply loosely. Anyone with a cough is liable to get that diagnosis pinned on him. If the cough is stubborn and interferes with one's normal way of life, then it makes good sense to get the opinion of an expert in diseases of the lung.

If the bronchitis is of long duration, or if stubborn infection takes hold in the bronchial tubes, they may become weak and dilated and collect large amounts of mucus and pus. The patient suffering from bronchiectasis has a chronic cough and shortness of breath, and brings up much phlegm and blood-tinged sputum. Sometimes the diagnosis can be suspected because the patient has developed a foul-smelling breath.

The chest specialist will make X-ray studies that complement ordinary X-ray techniques. He will inject iodized oil to outline the bronchial tubes more distinctly so they become more visible under X rays. They show up as dilated tubes.

The treatment depends upon individual requirements. We usually tell the patient to quit smoking. We advise that he use postural drainage a few times daily (lying head down over the bed) to help gravity drain the pus from the lungs. Medicines to loosen phlegm are helpful; so are antibiotics.

But really stubborn bronchiectasis may require operation for removal of severely infected lung segments. Sad it is that so many thousands of persons with a chronic cough fill themselves up with bottles of ineffectual cough medicines, thinking they just have bronchitis or some heart weakness when the real trouble is bronchiectasis.

A common cause for the persistent cough that frightens the imaginary heart patient is tension. It is frequently called the nervous cough, which, I suppose, is as good as any diagnosis, provided complete studies have eliminated

122

organic disease in the heart, lungs, and elsewhere as the cause.

I remember a thin, Mr. Milquetoast type of man (a clerk in the city tax office) who came in all broken out from bromides.

"I take them for my tension," he said, "because they relieve me better than aspirin or tranquilizers. But I've been told to quit bromides because I've been swapping my fear of heart disease for complications in the skin and even in my brain.

"I know why I've been so distraught. The trouble is I can't stand my boss. I'm under his thumb every minute of my working day. He seems to like to pick on me in front of everyone else in the office. He's the one whose giving me a heavy heart."

Immediately I suggested he stop taking bromides. Many people buy these concoctions over the counter (they require no prescription), renew them without checking with their doctor, and gradually drift into a condition we call bromidism or poisoning due to an overdose of bromides.

In addition to pimples and other forms of skin eruption, they may cause severe toxicity of the nervous system, with delirium, change of personality, and convulsions. I ordered my patient to take large quantities of table salt, which often acts as an antidote. I also suggested a change of jobs.

In my experience, unconscious emotional conflict between boss and employee often produces symptoms of imaginary heart trouble: chest pain, heart skips, and extreme fatigue. I told my visitor that if he continued in his present unhappy working environment, all the tranquilizers and drugs in China would not help.

I have observed similar instances of incompatibility between people in an office or shop. Sometimes the prob-

123

lem can be completely resolved by arranging a heart-to-heart talk with the boss, who is often unaware he has been acting like an overbearing martinet. It is the patient, however, who must make the first move if the problem remains unresolved. If he fails to take positive action he must resign himself to continuing anxiety about his heart.

Recently a patient told me that she was completely frustrated. An attractive widow who needed to support herself and three small children, she was concerned about her health. As an office manager in a small firm, she dressed neatly, had a trim figure, and gave every appearance of being a successful business woman. Nevertheless, the worry lines in her face belied her apparent control of herself.

"I've been examined by three of the finest specialists in our city, friends and colleagues of my late husband who was a physician," she said. "All of them have given me an OK on my health. Everything is normal, according to them. Yet I continue to have these frequent attacks of dizziness and nervousness. But what frightens me most is this cough I have. I keep thinking it's heart disease because my husband died of heart trouble and coughed so much during the last few months of his illness.

"I eat well enough, sleep fitfully, don't overwork, but keep worrying about my heart. My only bad habit is that I smoke about thirty cigarettes a day. Can you possibly refer me to some good internist in our town? I'd feel better with another medical opinion. I'd rather be taken care of by someone who doesn't know me than by doctors who were friends of my husband. They mean well, but I think they have a tendency to categorize me as a hypochrondriac."

A few months later I received a call from her saying that she had lost her cough and other nervous symptoms.

124

She gave two reasons. One, she had quit smoking. Two, the new doctor to whom I had referred her discovered she was suffering from hypoglycemia. He put her on a high-protein diet that cut down on carbohydrates, and she now felt like the proverbial new woman.

I was especially grateful for her call, because I had read an interesting article the previous evening about how hypoglycemia often is associated with heavy smoking.

The medical story had appeared in the *Annals of Internal Medicine* and was written by Maxwell G. Berry, M.D., of Kansas City, Missouri. He reported seeing twenty-four patients with tobacco hypoglycemia since 1946. In order of frequency, here are the symptoms noted by these patients: nervousness, dizziness, fatigue, blind staggers, headache, fainting, and cough.

Dr. Berry made the diagnosis of hypoglycemia only in patients who met the following criteria:

1. The use of one or more packages of cigarettes a day (or the equivalent).

2. Symptoms compatible with the diagnosis of hypoglycemia.

3. Blood sugar below 55 mg per 100 cc., concurrent with the above symptoms.

4. Prompt relief by the ingestion or administration of glucose (sugar) at the time symptoms occurred.

5. Complete and permanent relief of symptoms with cessation of smoking.

If you have a cough which disturbs you so much you begin to believe that it may be due to heart failure, no antagonist you must overcome is greater than the apparently innocuous one we call smoking. Whether the tobacco initiates any disorder in your body or simply aggravates it is an academic question.

A truism is this: You can't be as healthy and symptomless with smoking as you can without smoking. Tobacco is the common enemy—especially for people anxious about their hearts (forgetting, for a while, the increasing fears about the effects of tobacco on the lungs).

Many people rationalize away their bad habits. They say of smoking, "I enjoy it so much, I am willing to gamble on cancer of the lungs or heart trouble thirty years from now. I may get hit with a truck today when I cross the street, even if I don't smoke."

One common excuse is this: "I smoke so I won't gain weight. I consider I'm paying a health premium because if I stop smoking I'll get fat, and anyone knows that being fat causes a lot of trouble."

Yet, according to Jean Mayer, Ph.D., D.Sc., of Boston, Massachusetts: "It is quite advantageous to stop smoking cigarettes even at the risk of gaining weight. A well-known statistician has said that he estimates it would take a weight gain of over 120 pounds to offset the effect on longevity of two packs of cigarettes a day."

I like the statement by Stanley Schor, Ph.D., director of the AMA Department of Biostatistics: "The prudent man will not allow himself to gain weight when giving up cigarettes, and if he died sooner than expected it will be too late to kick himself for losing some enjoyment out of life."

Nevertheless, people continue to smoke. Even though they are afraid of heart disease or something else, some self-destructive impulse keeps them from quitting the habit. Warnings do not seem to help as much as we'd like.

For example, in a study published in the *Journal of the American Medical Association,* Starr Ford, Jr., M.D., and Fred Ederer, M.A., found that a combination of educational campaigns, psychotherapy, and pharmacological

126

aids used in smoking treatment clinics have produced only temporary alteration of cigarette-smoking habits:

> The agents used as smoking deterrents include local anesthetics, astringents, anticholinergics, tranquilizers, stimulants and nicotine substitutes. Apparently none of them has an established place in the treatment of the tobacco habit . . . No single method of therapy for terminating the cigarette habit has proved strikingly effective.

Americans smoke about 500 billion cigarettes every year. By the twelfth grade 40 to 45 percent of children are smoking. In high school, one in every four boys smokes, and one in every eight girls. Sixty percent of American men use tobacco, as do 30 percent of American women.

I can't understand it. I can't get used to it. Is it masochism to aggravate a rasping cough by smoking? Or is it plain stupidity? If stupidity is the answer, I am nevertheless compassionate without reservation. Even the stupid are to be pitied.

Take a morning several months ago, for example. I was sitting in the reception room of a hospital waiting for another doctor. I tried to read but could not relax because in the chair next to me sat a man wracked by a prolonged coughing seizure; he kept on coughing without any letup for at least fifteen minutes. I offered to get him some water, but he said, "No, thanks." At the time of my offer he was chewing gum. "Thanks be," I said to myself, "at least, he isn't smoking."

But the next time I turned I found I was wrong. He was a smoker. I hadn't seen him pull out the cigarette and light it, but there he sat with a long butt between his fingers. The coughing almost shook him apart, but as he coughed you could sense that he was waiting for it to stop, not just for reasons of comfort, but so he could take another drag on his cigarette.

Sure enough, that is what happened. Between the wheezes of noisy inspiration and the efforts of prolonged expiration he would take a deep whiff, and dense smoke would issue from his nose and mouth. When I finally departed, I realized that here was another of the many persons who go about slowly destroying themselves. They do not all necessarily progress to cancer of the lungs. Chronic bronchitis and emphysema are bad enough. And let's not forget how excessive smoking affects the person with heart skips, shortness of breath, nervousness, and other symptoms who is already questioning the strength of his heart.

According to the U.S. Public Health Service, if all Americans were nonsmokers, there would be 12 million fewer cases of chronic illness. Smoking is related to the existence of 300,000 extra coronary conditions, one million extra cases of chronic bronchitis or emphysema, nearly two million extra cases of sinusitis, and more than one million extra cases of peptic ulcers.

But it is natural to throw off statistics, however convincing. Perhaps if more smokers knew about "smoke" itself, they might consider quitting the habit.

Smoke is a mixture of these products of combustion: minute particles of solids and ashes, various vaporized chemicals and a mixture of gases. With each breath you take in some nicotine and tars as well as a supply of carbon monoxide. Lately it has been discovered that the nitrogen dioxide in cigarette smoke is an important contributory cause of emphysema. Think of all this every time you suck on a cigarette and deeply inhale all these noxious concoctions.

Oddly enough, many people resent the continued admonitions of physicians against smoking. Only recently a sixty-four-year-old neighbor of mine complained to me, "Why don't you let us live our own lives? I like to smoke and I'll keep on, cough or no cough. The trouble is that the modern doctor has learned too much. Too much about how cigarettes are bad for the heart or lungs or nerves. Years ago doctors didn't issue so many *don'ts.* I know you mean well. But let us live and die as we please. Oh, for the good old days!"

How pleasant it is to dream of the good old days. Peering through a multicolored spectrum that distorts the images of the past, we long for the horse-and-buggy days which seem so rosy-hued. But, except for the "boom of the bomb" which menaces us out there somewhere, I think most of us prefer the present to the past.

Especially is this true where medical care is in question. Recently I read an article by Williman L. Gould, M.D., written for the *New York State General Practice News,* which, I think, will interest you:

> Imagine! Ten cents for a doctor's prescription! That is the way it was in Abraham Lincoln's time, about 100 years ago.
>
> But then a penny bought a lot: one (or two) eggs, a cup of coffee, a large hunk of candy or a soda. Doctors' prescriptions were common for 10 cents to 50 cents. Now a single pill or capsule costs this latter amount.
>
> A century ago a doctor charged 25 cents for an office visit and 50 cents for a house call (any hour). Or the doctor would receive his fee in trade: a peck of potatoes, a bushel of tomatoes, a hair cut, two quarts of warm milk direct from the cow, or if the bill was large, maybe a pig.
>
> A local health officer received $25 for three

129

months, the same for a school teacher. The hospital charged a dollar a day. A working man was paid about 87½ cents per 12-hour day or night.

This was also the age of rickets and deformities. Maternal mortality was high. Each infant born had to struggle just to survive. Each adult was lucky if he could live to the age of 40.

The great scourges were tuberculosis, pneumonia, typhoid fever, diphtheria, measles, scarlet fever, smallpox, mastoid and brain abscess, meningitis, and many other infections too numerous to mention, but all conquered now.

Want to go back to the "good old days"? Would you exchange the penny prescriptions of yesteryear for the dollar ones of today? Would you trade modern wonder drugs for old-fashioned, homespun medicaments?

Perhaps it's true that the doctors of a few years ago were more permissive. If you smoked, OK. If you drank, OK. If you worked too hard, relaxed little, and overate, OK. There were few doctors and fewer organizations such as the cancer and heart societies of today to keep goading us on to live longer. Even now we choose to die in peace, to live in peace.

I suppose I could say, like an exasperated parent, "All right, cough your head off if you want to!" But preventive medicine is too ingrained in my system. I keep coming off the floor to take more blows from the insensitive who want to live without restrictions. Just as many resent the police when they try to enforce law and order, so many, who should know better, resent doctors who try to keep them healthy and alive.

8.

ACUTE INDIGESTION MAY
REALLY BE INDIGESTION

Indigestion is a wastebasket term. Into it we throw a varying number of symptoms in some way connected (we think) with an upset stomach or bowel. Each individual has his own definition of indigestion.

Maybe you take one martini too many at lunch and return to your office with a headache and an upset stomach. You call it indigestion.

You cannot withstand the urge to order lobster for dinner although you know quite well you are allergic to seafood and will have to pay the penalty: hives and an upset stomach. You call it indigestion.

Or you go to a party, famished, and actually destroy a platter of tidbits; drink too much bourbon, scotch or champagne; surround one or two helpings of steak or fried chicken (with the fixin's). You stuff yourself "up to here." You are awakened that night by a rebellious stomach, and the next day tell your associates, "Did I have a case of indigestion last night!"

But there are organic reasons, too, for a recalcitrant stomach. An ulcer can upset you. So can gall bladder trouble, chronic pancreatitis, kidney disease, hiatal hernia (mentioned in a previous chapter), ulceration of the bowel, cancer and scores of other conditions that cause the stomach and intestines to cry out with symptoms we label "indigestion."

For example, consider heart disease. Those old enough to remember are familiar with the frequent notices in the newspapers of reference to "acute indigestion":

> Mr. John Smith, well-known civic leader and industrialist, died of acute indigestion at home last night. He was apparently well when he came home from his office.
>
> Mrs. Adam Brown, wife of a prominent local attorney, suffered a sudden attack of acute indigestion yesterday. She is now a patient at the local hospital, in serious condition.

In the "good old days" the stomach was blamed for nearly everything. But the pendulum has a way of swinging widely through the years. Slowly less and less appeared in the newspapers about acute indigestion, and more and more about heart attacks. Progress in diagnosis with the aid of X rays and electrocardiograms was quickly rubbing out the term "acute indigestion" as the reason for sudden tragedies. At last, we knew that what seemed to be trouble with the stomach was often due to a weakened heart.

Soon people became aware that every stomach upset must be treated with respect. Any acute attack of "gas under the chest" accompanied by severe pain, nausea, and vomiting might, in fact, be due to a weakening heart muscle in which coronary arteries were unable to supply sufficient fuel so it could keep beating normally. Patients would send for their doctors, suspecting that what seemed like an ordinary stomach upset might really be due to a heart attack.

But, as often happens, the pendulum can swing too far. Although it is essential for one's well-being and very existence to keep alert to the possible masking of a heart attack by indigestion, this, too, can be overdone.

Every heart attack is not accompanied by symptoms of indigestion; and every attack of indigestion—acute or chronic—is not due to heart disease. Trouble in many other organs often simulates trouble in the heart. Correct diagnosis is imperative.

Gallstone trouble can fool the doctor and the patient if the diagnosis is not made early. For example, it is possible for a small stone to block a bile duct and cause extreme jaundice, without causing any pain. When this happens, the painless jaundice simulates a cancer in this region. What a relief when the surgeon finds that a gallstone is the troublemaker.

When gallstones or an otherwise functionless gall bladder cause chest pain, it is not unusual for the chronic pain or the acute distress to resemble that caused by coronary disease. Likewise, gall bladder disease is often mistaken for a stomach or duodenal ulcer, hiatal hernia, pancreatitis, arthritis of the spine (because of the referred pain between the shoulder blades), angina pectoris, and other conditions.

You might say, "Why all the difficulty? Isn't it easy to take gall-bladder X rays?" Easy, yes. But often the patient suffers for months or years before he goes to the doctor for a diagnosis. And even when he is seen early, the actual diagnosis may not be easy. Sometimes several X rays are necessary before trouble in the gall bladder can be accurately determined.

133

However, even after the definite diagnosis, the question of proper treatment is often raised. The patient asks himself, and his doctor, "Shall I or shall I not undergo surgery, now that I feel fine and the gallstone colic I had is a thing of the past?"

For example, a woman consulted me sometime ago about her husband who was under the care of another physician. "This past spring," she said, "my husband had pain in his chest. Our doctor put him in the hospital for a week thinking it might be his heart. But after special tests and X rays, he found some small gallstones.

"The doctor recommended surgery. My husband agreed to have it done a few months later. He went on a fat-free diet and so far has had no indigestion or chest pains. He is fifty-eight, a carpenter by trade, otherwise healthy—he has lost all his fears of having heart trouble—and is now wondering if he should submit to the knife."

She waited almost breathlessly for my reply. The situation she had described was not unusual but my experience had taught me the safest and most sensible procedure to follow under the circumstances.

"Your husband is in a common predicament," I told her. "The patient gets over his original attack of severe pain, has no subsequent indigestion or referred chest pains which worry him about his heart, and now wonders what all the shouting is about. He says: 'Suppose there are stones? Let them be. Let sleeping dogs lie. Why risk major surgery?' "

"That's exactly how my husband feels about it," she said.

"Fair enough," I replied. "However, here is the consensus of present medical thinking of the problem. Both the medical man and the surgeon prefer to have a patient come to an operation in good condition.

134

"Your husband is now in that fortunate state—except for his stones. Although removal of the gall bladder is still considered major surgery, operative reports from all over the world indicate there is little danger in undergoing the operation when patients are in good health otherwise.

"Here is what your doctor doesn't want to happen—and what your husband will be gambling against, if he doesn't submit to surgery now. One of the small stones may get caught in a bile duct, causing extreme jaundice with infection of the bile ducts and the liver itself. The gall bladder may become gangrenous. In other words, what might have been a simple operation and recovery then becomes some sort of a toss-up. Personally, I have come to believe that the best time for gall bladder surgery (when definitely indicated) is long before any serious complications set in to turn a routine operation into one on which life and death hang in the balance. I assure you, I am not being overly dramatic. Surgery of choice usually turns out better than surgery of urgent necessity."

Within a week the man had his gall bladder removed —against his will but at his wife's insistence. He had a routine recovery and convalescence, and became a convert to early operations. "I've never felt better," he told me in a subsequent telephone conversation. "No chest pains. No indigestion. I can eat anything now."

Many people have "silent stones" which are discovered during routine physical checkup. They have no symptoms. "Shall I have my gall bladder out?" they ask. Most doctors believe the answer should be yes.

Some patients, of course, insist on gambling. They feel well, so why submit to an operation? I have known many patients to live into their seventies and eighties with gallstones who never had any symptoms at all. One of my patients, who had had a bladder full of stones since the age of sixty, had an attack of colic while visiting in New Orleans at the age of eighty. She had the operation, an uneventful recovery, and lived to be ninety-five. Nevertheless, it is understandable that most older patients do not withstand gall bladder surgery as well as the younger group. I am hedging in my advice, because only the patient's personal physician can make the proper decision.

Consider this case history right out of the mouth of a fellow colleague. An excellent diagnostician, he told me the story of his wife's dilemma, undiagnosed for many years, during the course of a social visit to my home in Coral Gables, Florida:

"It all began one day while we were driving to New York City a number of years ago. At the time my wife was thirty-eight. When we were halfway to the city, she suddenly turned pale, reached over and said, 'Do you mind drawing to the side of the road? I feel nauseated." I helped her out of the car and we walked off the roadside into a pasture, where she vomited and felt immediately relieved. We returned to the car and passed it off as indigestion due to something she had eaten the previous night. Our stay in New York was uneventful.

"At no time during the next few months did she ever complain again. Then one night while we were visiting some friends at a dinner party, I looked across the room and noticed she was pale and looking faint. She asked me to take her home without telling our hostess that she was nauseated (not a fit compliment from a dinner guest). On the way home she informed me that she not only had nausea, but something new—a pressure under her chest. 'It feels like gas won't come up,' she said.

"When we got home she said, 'I don't like these attacks. I've also had a few more I didn't tell you about while you were busy in the office. Don't you think you ought to put me in the hospital for study? Frankly, I'm beginning to worry that I may have something wrong with my heart.'

"She went in for almost a week. I had the best cardiologist and the best gastroenterologist I know take care of her. X rays of her gall bladder and of her GI tract were negative. The three of us sat down to talk it over. Each man was positive that the heart and gall bladder (and all other organs) were in good working order. Diagnosis? They hated to make it, they said, but my wife was a victim of nerves. Only nervous upset could explain these frequent attacks.

"When my wife asked me for the final opinion, she was disappointed by the diagnosis. She said, 'John, you know I'm not the nervous type. Besides, you also know I'm under no mental strain of any kind. I still think it's my heart, even though X rays and ECG's are all right. You'll see; someday I'll be vindicated when I really have a severe heart attack."

At this point in his story, my doctor friend threw up his hands and shrugged his shoulders as if to say, "What does a doctor do in a case like this? He's more helpless than a layman when he has his own family to treat."

Then he resumed. "My recollection is that she had at least a dozen such attacks over a period of two or three months. Repeated ECG's and gall-bladder X rays kept coming back negative. I began to wonder, myself, if I didn't have a neurotic wife on my hands, in spite of her protestations that she was not tense or nervous about anything.

"Over the next ten years her attacks became less frequent. Nevertheless, she was in and out of my colleagues' offices getting check-ups and reassurance. She had a gall bladder X ray at least once every two years. The gall bladder always filled normally, there was good visualization and contraction after a fatty meal, and there was absolutely no evidence of stones.

"Now here comes the punch line. One day she was waiting for me in the lobby of New York's Hotel Plaza. I had left her for a few minutes to pick up a package and park the car for the day. When I entered the lobby, I noticed a small crowd standing around someone sitting in a chair in the corner. When I got closer, I saw it was my wife.

"She was perspiring profusely, hand over her left chest, pulse racing away with itself—the typical picture of a patient suffering a heart attack. They had picked her off the lobby floor.

"I immediately called an ambulance and notified a colleague who was an attending physician at his hospital. He examined her while she was still in the emergency room, then ordered an electrocardiogram. Although the first tracing was negative, he advised that she stay in emergency where she remained at least three hours before being wheeled into her own room.

"Both her doctor and I were now convinced that we were dealing with an organic heart patient. I thought to myself, 'She was right all the time. She's a coronary patient if I ever saw one.'

"But it was the same old story. Repeated ECG's daily for ten days were negative. So were the blood-enzyme tests. The doctor repeated a gall bladder examination, which was negative as usual. He discharged her at the end of two weeks.

"Now I come to the end of the story. One night about twenty years after the original attack, and about two weeks after a recent attack (with the usual negative ECG's and gall bladder X rays) she woke me because of ex-

138

treme chest pains referred down her arm and insisted she wanted to go to the hospital right away. 'This time,' she said, 'I know you'll find something is really wrong.'

"Electrocardiograms again proved negative. Then came a surprise! The radiologist's report the next day showed that she had a diseased gall bladder, and that four fairly large stones could be visualized on the X-ray film.

"You never saw any patient with gallstones so happy to learn the news. She was operated on two days later.

"Remember, now, that she had been suffering for more than twenty years as the wife of a supposedly good diagnostician. All of us had consigned her to the category of a cardiac neurosis. I keep thinking of the truism that a doctor who treats himself (or his family) has a fool for a patient. *Himself,* not the patient!

"I learned a lot from my wife's experience. It has helped a number of my patients who had similar symptoms and repeatedly negative ECG's and gall bladder X rays. I have a feeling that her symptoms over these many years were always due to her gall bladder even though the X rays were repeatedly negative. Otherwise, why should she now be symptom-free? It's years since she had her gall bladder removed.

"When patients continue to complain of chest pain and live scared because they are certain that the cause is undiagnosed coronary disease, I insist on a gall-bladder X ray. If the first one is negative, I get in touch with the X-ray man personally and ask that he use any special X-ray techniques necessary to be sure that there is no question that the gall bladder is absolved."

He turned to me with a rueful smile and said, "How do you feel about it?"

I told him I was hearing an echo of my own thoughts and beliefs. The gall bladder can be the great masquerader

139

when there is a question of the presence of heart disease. I focus upon it diagnostically until I get my answer.

I do not send a complaining patient out of my office with a diagnosis of "neurotic" until I have convinced myself completely that there is not one iota of evidence pointing to some organic disturbance elsewhere. Besides, many a so-called neurotic is cured of his belief that he has heart pains once his gall bladder is removed.

Not only patients with attacks of acute gallstone colic resemble those with coronary disease; so do those who have a chronic, nonfunctioning gall bladder (with or without stones).

Many a patient has become apprehensive about some heart weakness because he has had such complaints as heartburn, pressure of gas under the chest, "heaviness around the heart" after meals, and a dull ache between the shoulder blades.

What a frustrating feeling for both doctor and patient (mostly for the patient) not to be able to have a definite diagnosis. It leaves you hanging in midair, wondering when something is going to cut you down. Unfortunately, symptoms do not invariably fit into one neat, diagnostic package. Many diseases leave us in the dark. Not until months or years later—as in the case of the wife of my colleague—are we able to make a positive diagnosis.

Nevertheless, it is true that usually the diagnosis is right there for the asking if we look hard enough.

Concerned individuals often ask, "Who is the best heart specialist in the United States? My husband has been bothered by chest pains and indigestion quite often. He's worried about his heart. Our family doctor diagnosed his condition as nerves due to business tension. Although we have great confidence in our family doctor, we want the best. Money is no object. After all, it's his life!"

140

My answer is to tell them that, though distance may lend enchantment where "specialists" are concerned, it is no guarantee of greater ability in the medical practitioner involved. Your own family doctor, around the corner, may turn out to be the best doctor in the country for your husband. The family doctor knows his weaknesses and his strengths, his idiosyncrasies and his fears.

These days the well-trained general practitioner can make a diagnosis of coronary disease and knows the established treatment. If any question arises in management —when to get out of bed and the use of blood thinners, for example—the good family doctor will ask for consultation with a heart specialist. And he may be quite a good specialist, even though he works in the same city and your husband doesn't have to travel hundreds of miles for an examination and opinion. And if you live in a large city it is likely one of your hospitals has a coronary care unit where he will receive the most modern attention, if his trouble is coronary disease.

Not only elderly people but young-marrieds often are concerned about their hearts. Indigestion, they believe, is the cloak that hides their heart failure. Health, of course, is problem number one—as it is for everyone, regardless of age. But I am convinced that most young husbands and wives who have shoved off in their little skiff on the high seas of matrimony will agree that financial problems are high on the list of storm threats to their marriage craft.

Worry about how to make the proverbial ends meet is the daily ingredient of unhappiness and disagreements. Some wives say, "My husband is too lazy. He has no ambition." Others complain, "I wish John wouldn't be so ambitious. He works so hard I'm worried about his health."

Here is an example of the latter complaint. It came

141

from a pretty young suburban housewife, a woman who was very sensible in her outlook on life and justifiably concerned about her marriage mate.

"My husband is twenty-nine and I am twenty-four," she said. "We have three children. I would be the happiest woman if he would only be contented. Instead, he is too ambitious. And I think he's paying for it already. He complains of indigestion every day. Once he admitted to me, and it worried me because he is so close-mouthed, that he wondered if the trouble was really in his heart.

"He has taken on a second job. He is moonlighting and works about eighteen hours a day. We used to be a happy family, but we rarely see him anymore. He works as a telephone repairman during the day. All he comes home for is to have a hasty dinner and rush out to his second job at our local post office. He says he's doing it for all of us. And he keeps taking pills for his indigestion and his heart.

"He seems to have some kind of insecurity because his parents were poor. 'I don't want our kids to go through what I did,' he keeps on saying, 'and I don't want you to have to worry like my mother did.'

"Believe me I appreciate what he is trying to do, but I think he'll get sick if he keeps on. He has lost weight, he is very nervous and jumpy, and is already beginning to look sick. He has been complaining of stomach pains more and more. I wish I could get him into your office for an examination and some advice."

I told her she might have a difficult time in getting him to visit me. Some men are stubborn. They don't give in until they are jolted by sudden illness. The trouble is the young think that youth itself protects them from any severe complications. They do not realize that continued strain, day in and day out, at last takes its retribution—whatever the age of the person involved.

I told her about an overly ambitious young man like her husband, who took on two jobs so he could pay for his last year of college. He was studying for a Ph.D. Anyone will admit this is a commendable ambition. But in his case it proved to be more than he could handle. At the age of twenty-seven he suffered severe hemorrhages from a bleeding ulcer. Fortunately, he survived, but there was no doubt that life's daily pressures almost contributed to an early death.

I suggested that she keep nagging her husband into having an examination, The fact that he didn't look well, was losing weight, was nervous, had stomach pains (and was worried about his heart) were sufficient reasons for believing that "something isn't right somewhere."

"If he comes in," I said, "I think he will see the entire picture more clearly. Even if he makes extra money to give him security, it is likely that most of it will vanish in a pile-high stack of doctor and hospital bills.

"Moonlighting may be all right occasionally for a few weeks or months. But when carried on for years just to make more money it can become a serious threat to health and life.

"High blood pressure, diabetes, hyperthyroidism, heart disease, ulcers, and many other illnesses rub their hands greedily, figuratively speaking, and wait around the corner to pounce on the man who becomes overambitious."

The persuasive power of a woman is something to contemplate. Within a week the husband appeared for his examination. First, I listened and learned that he was, indeed, anxious about his heart. He had kept his real fears from his wife. One reason he worked so hard was to "make more" so he could leave more if he had a heart attack. His examination proved negative. You never saw a more thankful patient. He gave up his second job. And their life together gradually became more serene and sensible.

Another form of indigestion which mimics heart disease is ulcer of the stomach or duodenum. Pain can be nagging and bearable or so excruciating that a patient may have to be rushed to the hospital.

In the first instance, a chronic eroding ulcer causes heartburn, recurring pains, gas, pressure under the lower chest and upper abdomen. Sometimes pains shoot up the left chest "over the heart."

In the second instance, and relatively rare, is the sudden, acute pain which is so intense it throws the patient into shock. It is sometimes mistaken for an actual coronary attack. There is vomiting, the patient writhes in discomfort, and his belly becomes as hard as a board. His life depends upon early diagnosis. If operated on within an hour or two, most patients with perforation due to ulcer recover.

But it is the diagnosis that is so important.

Once I was asked for my list of the ten worst habits a person can have. I believe anyone can make up an entirely different list and still be right. But here are mine, and not in the order of their importance: 1. Smoking. 2. Overdrinking. 3. Overeating (obesity). 4. Underexercising or overexercising. 5. Undervacationing. 6. Undersleeping (too many cheat on sleep by watching the late-late show). 7. Harboring resentment. 8. Worrying unnecessarily. 9. Living in tension at work and at home. 10. Self-treatment and procrastination.

Let us consider numbers 8 and 10. They really tie

144

in together. When you treat yourself you stay away from the doctor. And not knowing just what you suffer from, it is likely that you worry about yourself.

Often there is still time to stop smoking, drinking, living in tension, and quitting any of the other bad habits, but procrastination keeps a person worrying for weeks, months and years unnecessarily. And if real disease is present, sometimes it doesn't give a second chance.

The day has long passed when people wear the badge of ulcer with pride. As with gout, there is no longer any "status" connected with stomach ulcer. Years ago only kings, dukes, and the very wealthy were supposed to be susceptible to such an affliction as gout. Now we know that the carpenter who repairs the roof of the palace and the plumber who repairs the pipes—as well as the doctor who treats the high-and-mighty—can come down with the gout, too.

And so it is with ulcers. It is not where you live (Hollywood or New York are the supposed ulcer capitals of the United States) but what you are that determines whether you will suffer from ulcers.

In my experience I have found ulcer patients to be typically tense, keen, overemotional, hard-working individuals. They are the ones most likely to translate an ulcer pain into heart pain. Many come in first complaining of heart trouble rather than of stomach trouble.

There has been some question lately whether top executives are more prone to ulcer than others. Some evidence indicates they have less such trouble than their employees. This is understandable.

Those on the lower rungs, climbing up, necessarily have their hands stepped on occasionally—and this produces resentment and animosity. These characteristics are like gasoline for the fire of an ulcer. They light up symptoms that extend into the chest and put the fear of heart disease into some of these patients.

Although it is evident that in the care of an ulcer you will have better chance of improvement if you follow your doctor's directions concerning diet and medication, there are other important considerations. You must learn how to come to terms with yourself as a person—and with the people in your environment. This means getting along at the office or shop or at home with the human beings you find there.

Don't expect any of them to be perfect—neither are you. Remember that an ulcer feeds on tension and resentment, and that relaxation and peace of mind favor healing (and prevention). The sooner an ulcer is brought under control, the sooner will apprehensions about having heart disease vanish because of referred pains in the chest.

One of the worst ulcers I ever had to deal with was in a barber who hated the man who worked next to him. He almost bled to death on three occasions, and had a total of thirty blood transfusions. Not until he came to terms with himself and with the man he once hated (they are happy partners in business now) did his ulcer heal and his chest pains disappear.

Another bad one was in a young farm boy who came to me complaining of chest pains and was sure he had heart disease. But an examination showed he had a duodenal ulcer. This boy had been promised a college education by his father. When the showdown came, the father used every kind of excuse (including feigned illness) to keep his son as a helper on the farm.

For two years the youngster stewed in hatred against his father for letting him down. He almost died, too. Not until the father learned that he was the cause, and relented, did the boy recover. He is now a successful attorney.

Although it is true that we do not know the actual cause of ulcers of stomach and duodenum, there is no question that emotional stress, especially if prolonged for months and years, can aggravate an existing ulcer—if not cause it.

If an ulcer is the reason for the chest pains you thought were due to heart disease, don't blame yourself. Somewhere inside you are the twists and turns and pulls of emotion which either give you a contented stomach and psyche, or cause it to boil up into an ulcer or two. Reasons vary.

For example, after a lecture in Detroit a few years ago, a distinguished-looking man, heavy-set and about six foot two, came up to the platform to congratulate me because I had brought home a point with which he was personally familiar.

"I had chest discomfort at first, which I surely thought was due to heart disease. Although doctors found I had an ulcer, I was relieved to know the cause of the pains. You'll never guess how and why I developed the ulcer. Well, this may interest you."

He stopped a moment, smiling in memory of his experience, then continued. "My personal life is as satisfactory as any man can wish for. I am president of a successful company, with capable executives who carry the load efficiently. I have a wonderful wife, five children and twelve grandchildren.

"Until the past few years, I have been what you might define as the happy man. But when I began to experience a gnawing sensation in the pit of my stomach. I won't keep you in suspense any longer. What's really eating me is the good American taxpayers' money the government keeps sending out to 'keep friends' and 'make friends.'

"I almost had a relapse the other day when I read that we had the gall or foolhardiness (whatever you choose to call it) to send another few million dollars to Tito—within days after he publicly sided with Russia on the Cuban problem, and was on his way to Moscow to receive a few bear hugs from the Premier himself. That adds up, I understand, to about three billion dollars we have given an enemy like Tito on a platter.

"I wish I could use four-letter words and temper outbursts to relieve my feelings on this matter. The trouble is that I keep these feelings to myself. But after hearing your talk on the need for not bottling up resentments, I'm turning over a new leaf."

I recall sitting next to a philosophical-minded dinner partner. She was a patient whose family I had treated for years. Although over fifty she had the charm and enthusiasm of a woman in her thirties. Her pepper-and-salt hair was artfully arranged and her smiling eyes and well-preserved features mirrored the vitality that animated all her actions.

She said, "I am one of those who don't take things for granted. I continue to marvel at the wonders of the human body. I suppose this is not the time, at a dinner party, to become physiological, but I think most of us forget. For example, our hand goes to our mouth with a morsel of food, we chew, we swallow, and then forget about it. Think of all that must go on within the body to digest and assimilate the food. It makes one glad to be alive."

As a doctor, of course I agreed. And I told her there was no need to make any excuses for becoming physiological at a dinner party. I said, "The body is a busy, chemical plant. Let's follow the course of that morsel of food. Our teeth grind it to a pulp. The tongue helps, as it is a strong muscle bundle itself. While this bolus of food is still in the mouth the salivary glands go into action. The salivary juice acts predominantly on the starches in the food, converting it into carbohydrates. Other enzymes break down these carbohydrates into simpler molecules of sugar.

"At the moment of swallowing, the epiglottis seals off the top of the windpipe so food won't go down the wrong way. After the food enters the esophagus, the peristaltic action of its muscles propels it into the stomach."

I stopped, looked at her and asked, "Am I spoiling your appetite for all this delicious food you have here. Tell me and I'll stop. After all, you started it, and have the right to call it off."

She smiled graciously and shook her head. "No, go right ahead. I'm having fun."

So I continued in this elementary lesson in physiology.

"The powerful muscles in the stomach then grind the food into smaller particles. Its tiny gastric glands secrete many enzymes and hydrochloric acid. For example, one enzyme curdles milk, another splits the fats, and still another works on the proteins.

"In three to five hours, the meal, which has been changed to a semifluid mass called chyme, passes into the small intestine. This is about twenty feet long (four times as long as the large intestine). More digestive juices mix with the food as it enters the first part of the intestine which we call the duodenum. These secreted by the pancreas and the liver.

"Proteins are further broken down into amino acids, carbohydrates into simpler sugars, and fats into fatty acids. Bile also helps to emulsify fats and prepare them for absorption.

149

"Farther down in the small intestine are millions of microscopic villi whose job it is to absorb water and the final products of digestion. The blood vessels carry the food products to the liver which processes the carbohydrates, absorbs the fats, and acts as a storehouse for vitamins, minerals, and iron. When the remains of the food leave the small intestine and enter the large bowel, they become the waste, semisolid material that is eliminated later."

I paused a moment, then added, "You are probably tired of taking this technical journey, but let me point out that your stomach, intestines, liver, pancreas, and all the rest are uncomplaining. Day after day, while you are awake and while you sleep, this intricate factory is on a twenty-four-hour shift.

"Therefore, we doctors say that when there are complaints, it is better to heed them before the machinery breaks down. Heartburn, gas, abdominal or chest pain, jaundice, loss of appetite, constipation, diarrhea—these are indications that an organ is working under difficulty and is in danger of going on strike.

"The sooner you take the trouble to your doctor, the more likely will you get an early, satisfactory settlement. Removal of gallstones and a faulty gall bladder, treatment of an ulcer, or of trouble in the liver, pancreas, esophagus, or large intestine—these are the usual ways to placate a complaining gastrointestinal system.

"That's the end of the lecture," I informed her. "But I suppose I don't have to remind you, because of your husband's personal experience, that his 'heart attack' fortunately turned out to be due to a hiatal hernia. If he hadn't come in early for diagnosis, he'd still be worrying that the pains in his chest are heart pains. We can be thankful he didn't become a cardiophobe."

150

Another commonly overlooked condition that occasionally produces chest discomforts and fear of heart disease is pancreatitis. In its chronic form it can produce indigestion similar to that found in chronic gall bladder disease, hiatal hernia, ulcer, chronic gastritis. In its acute attack, it can produce as much pain and shock as an actual attack of coronary thrombosis.

When all kinds of X rays and other tests keep coming back negative in a patient who continues to complain of indigestion, the doctor should take special tests to check pancreatic function.

Of course, acute gastritis itself simulates the "acute indigestion" often found during a heart attack. As many may know, acute gastritis is the formal name for a rather common ailment that goes by the name of upset stomach. The causes are many. Fever alone can do it. It can be a part of symptoms of serious illness such as failing kidneys or hepatitis.

Ordinarily an uncomplaining organ, the stomach occasionally reminds us that it doesn't like to be taken for granted and kicks over the traces when least expected. For example, you may be a habitual overeater and get away with it ninety-nine times out of a hundred. But there comes the time when the stomach may show its resentment at being overloaded by reacting with symptoms of nausea, vomiting, pain in the upper abdomen and chest. Sometimes the intestines join in the revolt, and the patient also has diarrhea.

In like manner, oversmoking may occasionally cause acute gastritis; more commonly, so may too many alcoholic drinks. There are times when the walls of the stomach and intestines flinch at a certain food to which they are allergic. So the stomach and intestines try to expel it. The same situation holds true with tainted foods. Some people with especially sensitive stomachs get acute gastritis if they drink ice water; others suffer from an upset stomach when they take simple medicines that have no adverse effect on other people.

The basic treatment is simple: Give the overburdened or insulted stomach a rest. Fasting for at least a day, taking occasional hot tea and dry toast, is often a successful treatment.

Simple, acute gastritis should not last more than a few hours. If stomach pain, nausea, vomiting, and chest pain persist, don't go through another day without seeking medical assistance.

In these days when man has the opportunity to live several years longer than did his ancestors at the turn of the century, each one of us must develop his own philosophy of aging. Some of us feel ancient at forty (especially on that birthday) while others go their merry way ignoring the calendar years.

9.

HEART MURMURS
ARE OFTEN MEANINGLESS

Take this to heart: you may have a murmur and *not* have heart disease: you may have heart disease and *not* have a murmur.

Undoubtedly, the heart is the seat of life. When it loses its function as an efficient pump to propel blood to all the tissues of the body, then the brain, lungs, liver, kidneys, and all the rest of the organs suffer.

Therefore, it is natural for people to become upset and fearful when they learn that they have a heart murmur. For years doctors have been saying that all murmurs are not a threat to health or life. We have said that functional murmurs are of no importance. Even organic murmurs (where there is actual damage to a heart valve) vary in their severity.

For example, many thousands of women with murmurs due to rheumatic heart disease are able to have babies and raise families, and men with such murmurs are able to pursue their vocations. Therefore, if you know you have a murmur and are concerned about it, have your family doctor and a cardiologist evaluate its importance. Don't

153

go through life wondering whether you have heart disease.

Here is an encouraging letter I recently received from one of the readers of my newspaper column:

> What I say may help others, if you repeat it. When I was a child I had rheumatic fever and several other illnesses. What has always stayed in my mind was the fact that I had developed a heart murmur due to rheumatic fever. Doctors told my parents that I would never be able to bear children unless I took good care of myself. Well, here I am, married nearly twenty-one years, the mother of five children. The youngest is three, the oldest is twenty.
>
> My mother and dad carried this fear of my murmur for many years and then told me about it after my first child was born. I went to a heart specialist who told me the murmur wasn't important. My history certainly proves it. My reason for telling you about myself is to put parents of such children at ease. All my children are as healthy as can be. You must know that a mother raising a family of five children goes through stresses and strains. So I hope that worried people see that all heart murmurs may not be as bad as they think they are.

There are murmurs and murmurs—the functional ones (of absolutely no threat to health) and the organic, which are a part of actual heart disease. But in the minds of the worrisome, these are all lumped together as threats to existence.

Dr. Chester P. Lynxwiler and Dr. James L. Donahue of St. Louis discovered that innocent heart murmurs in children are quite common. They found such murmurs in 36 percent of 1,706 children. The murmur disappeared or remained in the innocent category in 97.5 percent of the

154

patients observed over a period of six years. They discovered that the incidence of innocent murmurs was highest between the ages of eight and twelve.

Whether it is real or functional, just what is a murmur? It is a sound caused by the swirl and swish of blood currents as they pass over the valves of the heart or over blood vessel walls that are roughened. You might liken a faint murmur to that produced by water as it gently trickles over small pebbles in a quiet valley rivulet; while a loud, strident murmur would be similar to one produced by a torrent of water falling over large rocks in a mountain stream.

I believe that no physician—especially an insurance examiner who doesn't know his patient intimately—should ever tell a person, "You have a murmur," unless he has completed an extensive diagnostic survey. Even then, it may not be necessary to so inform the patient of what has no real significance.

Several of my colleagues have confessed that the only reason they do not keep this knowledge from patients is because of sad experiences in the past. As one said, "I always say there is a murmur when I have found it. I do not keep it from the patient, even though he may become scared. My reason? Sometime in the future, another doctor may examine him and say, 'You have a murmur.' The patient will return, angry, and ask, 'Why did you keep it from me? I was entitled to know.' Therefore, I feel it is my duty to tell."

I disagree. It is a doctor's duty *not to tell* if the patient has a functional murmur. Otherwise, the patient may develop iatrogenic heart trouble (of which I wrote in an earlier chapter). He may live in needless fear for the rest of his life.

Dr. Edward Weiss had some interesting and reassuring

155

remarks to make about murmurs in Philadelphia a number of years ago where he appeared as a faculty member at a postgraduate heart seminar. I attended and was impressed by his unique understanding of the human being and his emotions. The following excerpts from his remarks have particular pertinence:

> Probably no single objective finding leads to more false diagnoses of cardiac disease than a murmur. A systolic murmur can be found in a large number of healthy young adults if they are examined in various postures, in different phases of respiration, before and after exercise. These functional murmurs are also much more common during fever. They are rather faint, but sometimes moderately loud, and are heard in the apical or pulmonic areas. . . .
>
> If there is any question regarding the significance of the murmur the patient had better not be apprised of the fact or even be made suspicious of heart disease until one can marshal his evidence in order completely to exonerate the heart. . . .
>
> The beginning of a cardiac neurosis can often be traced to the indiscreet remark of the examining physician who detects for the first time a systolic murmur at the apex of the heart unaccompanied by other evidence of organic disease.

Once this seed of anxiety is planted it often takes deep root. For years later, reassuring opinions by dozens of other competent cardiologists may be unable to convince the patient that the functional murmur is unimportant. All he remembers is the awful verdict he heard years ago: "You have a heart murmur."

I recall a young married man, recently graduated from college, who came in one day for a heart checkup:

"I'm a miserable guy," he said. "Here I am with everything to live for, a nice wife and a strapping six-month-old son, and I've just learned I have a murmur. As you know, I'm a copywriter with an ad agency and I've come right from the office of an insurance examiner who gave me the bad news. I came here on the same day because I want to know the truth about my heart before I get home tonight."

I had known this young man since he was a child. He was handsome, tall, with good solid shoulders, thick black hair, fine features, and a sunny disposition. On and off over the years I had heard a faint murmur, brought on by rapid heart action due to exercise tests in my office. After fifteen minutes it would disappear entirely. (It seems that our young man had run up a few flights of stairs to the insurance examiner, and had reproduced the same murmur I had heard after exertion on his part).

I had never told him he had a murmur because it was undoubtedly functional and not due to heart disease. Had I done so, this four-letter man in high school and well-known college athlete might have been too frightened even to pedal a bike down the street.

Now as I examined him, his heart was racing with fright, and the faint murmur was present. But X rays, electrocardiograms, and other tests proved that he still was free from organic heart disease. Having been his family doctor for so long, I was able to convince him that he was perfectly healthy. But it took a lot of doing. I spent at least an hour explaining to him that there are all kinds of murmurs, and that most of them are functional and of no consequence.

However, if a physician does find actual heart disease and a murmur tied in with it, the patient should be in-

157

formed. I am just as insistent that a person with a functional heart murmur need *not* know, as I am that a heart patient *should* know.

If you have ever been told that you have a murmur, remember that it is either functional or real. The next step is to insist on a complete cardiac survey. Do not accept a simple, hurried "laying on of the stethoscope on the chest" for the ultimate diagnosis.

Too many lives have been curtailed by insufficient evidence. Too many have accepted, without confirmation, that they must live like semi-invalids because someone found they had a murmur.

Be sure you "have the works" in a specialist's office before you hang out the white flag of surrender. Too many are certain that they are approaching a state of rigor mortis when they learn they have a "heart leak." It is difficult for the healthy person to understand how much anguish another healthy person with a functional murmur can suffer.

The following letter from a frightened mother will give you some idea how much parents suffer when told that their child has a murmur:

> Please consider this letter and its contents as if I were sitting in your office talking to you. I could not face you, in person, and say what I am about to say because I would freeze with fear. Just thinking of my child's murmur sends me into a stony silence.
>
> It all began a few months ago when I took my three-year-old daughter, Jane, to a pediatrician for a vaccination. While we were there he put his stethoscope on her chest and nonchalantly said, "Oh, she seems to be all right, except that she might have a slight murmur."
>
> As my own brother has a rheumatic heart and his

158

first child was born with a defective heart valve and a murmur, I am sensitized to the word "murmur." I was so shocked at his words I almost fainted.

When the doctor saw how disturbed I was, he tried to comfort me by saying, "There's nothing actually wrong with your daughter's heart." I said to him, "If that's true, then why did you even have to mention the murmur if it wasn't important?" He shrugged his shoulders.

I couldn't wait until two days later when I had an appointment with a heart specialist. He put our little one through all the known modern tests. You can imagine how happy I was when he said that the slight murmur had no significance. I felt wonderful, and forgot about it until a few months later.

Our daughter was taken to a neighborhood clinic for some booster shots they recommended at her age. While she was there, a doctor who was examining her heart said, "Has she ever had rheumatic fever? She has a murmur!"

I actually staggered out of the clinic. I felt disgusted and depressed. It seemed that my child's murmur was following her around wherever she went. So, I took her back to the heart specialist. He examined her in at least a half-dozen different positions, before and after exercise.

He is a patient, kindly man. He said, "I'm glad to be able to tell you again that it's nothing. She has a functional murmur. Her heart is normal. Either you believe me, in spite of how many more times you hear about her murmur, or you'll go through life living scared—and making your daughter a cardiophobe, too."

Here you have one of many examples where needlessly and tactlessly informing a patient of a child's functional murmur set up a whirlpool of daily anxiety in the mind of the mother. We doctors must forever be aware against instilling unnecessary fears in our patients.

For some parents, learning that a child has a murmur (whatever its nature) is a shattering experience. I have seen many formerly stable and emotionally well-balanced parents go to pieces on hearing the news, especially when there seem to be some contradictions in the doctor's findings.

For example, one doctor will find a functional murmur and say, "It's unimportant. His heart is all right." Yet, his next words will be, "Just for safety's sake, better not let him play baseball or football or any other games that require a lot of physical exertion. Let's play it safe."

One woman, just returning from her doctor's office couldn't understand why her nine-year-old, quite active and apparently healthy, should have to give up sports. She could only reach the conclusion that her doctor thought the boy really had a bad heart. Otherwise, why did the doctor restrict his activities?

Doctors need to be extremely tactful with parents who show evidence of suffering from chronic anxiety about themselves or about family members. It is true, nevertheless, that doctors are not always to blame for instilling fear into these children or their parents. I have known patients so susceptible to anxiety that, no matter how tactfully I explained an innocuous, functional murmur, they would continue to live in apprehension.

Nevertheless, we must tell such a patient, "You have a strong heart; it's all in your head." We mustn't say, "You have only a slight deviation from the normal in your electrocardiogram." The proof of how the doctor really feels about his patient should be inherent in the following parting advice: "You do not have heart disease. Make full use of its power. You can do anything with it that anyone else can."

Some people's fears will disappear after one completely reassuring visit to an understanding doctor. Others, refusing to take their doctor's assurances on faith, become sufficiently psychoneurotic to require special psychosomatic management or help from a psychiatrist.

The latter case is often true in instances where people have suffered an unforgotten emotional shock while they were young.

As an architect patient of mine put it: "I've been suffering from what you call imaginary heart trouble since my dad died suddenly and unexpectedly over a dozen years ago. He had been told he had a murmur, but I had never asked what kind it was. Since then I've been scared because my own doctor detected a slight murmur in my heart a few months after my dad's death.

"Heart disease immediately became a bugaboo to me. The seed of fear had been planted in my mind. To water it, so to speak, a close friend of mine died of rheumatic heart disease about two years later. He also had murmurs.

"I became petrified. For the past ten years I've lived with the horrible fear I might drop dead suddenly. Nothing seems to help. Many doctors like you have been kind enough to examine me thoroughly and almost swear that my heart is all right, but I keep hearing the murmur, as if it were splashing about in my mind. Do you think a psychiatrist may help?"

In his case, it seemed advisable to see a psychiatrist. I am glad to say that after a year of patient treatment, he lost most of his earlier fears and returned to the mainstream of life a happier and better-adjusted person. Fortunately, most people with functional murmurs show

161

improvement after routine treatment by a sympathetic, understanding family doctor or cardiologist.

The couch is not a necessary adjunct of therapy for all persons who think they have heart disease. For some, statistics such as the following may bring them the comfort they need to live as unfrightened individuals:

In a recent article in *Today's Health,* "Heart Murmur —What Does It Mean?" Shirley Motter Linde quoted two interesting sources that indicate the unimportance of some murmurs.

In one study by Dr. William E. Morton and Dr. Leland A. Huhn, heart specialists of Denver, Colorado, more than 15,000 children were examined and 83 percent were found to have innocent heart murmurs. About half the murmurs could be heard at one examination, but not at a second one.

In another study by two Seattle pediatricians of ninety-three students who had been told they had a "bad heart," seventy-five of them were normal and yet thirty of the children were being restricted in activities, some of them even kept home from school.

E. S. Kilgore, M.D., wrote some time ago in the *Journal of the American Medical Association* as follows:

> If not very loud, if not high-pitched, if markedly changed by respiration and posture, and if not accompanied by other signs of heart disease (especially enlargement of the heart), by deficient heart function, or by a history of rheumatism or chorea, these systolic murmurs should not be regarded as pathologic.

Statistics are not always cold and impersonal. Like a friendly arm around one's shoulder, they can be heartening.

10.

OTHER REASONS
FOR ANKLE SWELLING

Swelling of the legs and ankles is a common symptom. For many people, it is frightening. Immediately they translate it into trouble with the heart or kidneys.

Although it is true that in congestive heart failure and in kidney disease leg swelling may be a symptom, it is important not to make quick guesses. Proper heart evaluation and routine examination of urine and blood will either convict or exonerate the heart or kidneys.

Sometimes the swelling (edema) is due to less anxiety-provoking factors. Recently I have run across a simple reason for leg swelling not connected with serious organic illness. The following abstract is from an article by Dr. Charles A. Ribaud and Dr. Anthony A. Formato in *Review of Modern Medicine:*

> The tourniquet effect of a tight-legged panty girdle which encases the thighs with elastic material can cause swelling of feet and ankles. Constriction of venuous and lymphatic return from the legs increases hydrostatic pressure, which will result in edema. Changing to another type of girdle corrected the condition in two patients.

Abnormal swelling of ankles or legs deserves complete investigation. Fortunately, the cause is not always a serious one.

Here, for example, is the case of a woman in her twenties who came to me, expressing considerable concern about a swelling problem.

"Until the past three weeks my weight has been about 118 pounds, but lately I have been gaining by bloating," she told me. "What bothers me most is that when my ankles swell I worry about my heart. My mother died of heart trouble and she had swollen ankles for months before she passed away.

"But my doctor says my heart is all right. My trouble is caused by hormonal imbalance. He has given me 'water shots and water pills.' Usually they take off about seven to nine pounds in a few days. Must I live on these pills daily to keep my bloating and ankle swelling down? I am almost scared to eat or drink anything. I keep thinking about my heart."

I told her that hormonal imbalance might do just that —cause excessive retention of fluid in the tissues and increase weight. In some women, swelling of the legs, bloating, and nervousness are a part of a syndrome we call premenstrual tension.

For years we could do nothing to relieve their discomforts. But now we can bring relief by prescribing a combination of tranquilizers, hormones, and diuretics (water pills) for about a week before the expected period.

For those suffering from bloating and swelling, doctors sometimes order diuretics for weeks instead of days. But I believe that patients should understand that this apparently simple method of removing excess fluid should not be taken lightly. Especially it should not be overdone during weight-reduction regimes. This may upset the min-

164

eral balance in the body. When large amounts of fluid are lost, sodium and potassium imbalance result. This may cause extreme weakness and nervousness.

Most doctors warn their patients against taking water pills without supervision for long periods of time. Rapid weight loss by use of diuretics, often repeated, can be potentially harmful. One precaution during such rapid weight loss due to diuretics is to build up the potassium in the blood by taking potassium as medicine and by eating such foods as fish, meat, molasses, prunes, raisins, almonds, spinach, peanuts, whole wheat, olives, or avocados.

Although this young woman continued to have monthly bloating and ankle swelling, well controlled by the methods I have just described, she soon lost all fear that she might have heart disease. A few weeks later she told me why.

"It came about when you asked me that question I couldn't answer. Remember, last month, when you said, 'Does it make sense that your heart should be well for three weeks of every month and then fail for one week before your period?' No, it didn't make sense and I stopped worrying about my heart."

Every day hundreds of thousands of frightened pseudo-cardiacs visit their doctors in the United States. In their own minds, heart disease is more than a shadowy, menacing specter; it is a reality.

If you have swelling of the ankles do not jump to the conclusion that you must have heart disease. Especially may this not be true if the swelling is an isolated complaint. In other words, such edema (in the presence of real heart disease) is usually accompanied by one or more other symptoms, such as shortness of breath, cough, indigestion, fatigue, and pain.

Nevertheless, you may also have these symptoms and

165

(as I have been saying throughout these pages) not have actual heart disease.

I remember a woman who had ankle swelling, cough, shortness of breath, indigestion, fatigue, pain—to repeat the common symptoms—yet had a strong heart. What caused her symptoms? She had a reason for each one of them.

She was a middle-aged woman about fifty pounds overweight. She told me that the ankle swelling occurred only when she was on her feet a lot during hot weather. Cool weather made it disappear. Her indigestion was due to a gall bladder filled with stones. Her cough, to cigarettes. Her shortness of breath to stairs and overweight. Her tiredness was the result of obesity and worry about her heart. Diet took off excess poundage and relieved her of shortness of breath and fatigue. She quit cigarettes and her cough vanished. Operation on her gall bladder removed her indigestion and occasional chest pain.

But the most important factor was that now she lived a life free from the constricting apprehensions brought on by fear of heart disease. She acknowledged that at last she believed what I had said months before, "Your heart is stronger than you think."

A fifty-year-old man came to my office one day, pointed to a swollen ankle, and said, "I knew some day I'd come down with heart trouble. Just look at that ankle. It has been puffy and swollen for months."

His legs had been covered with varicose veins for years. In the affected leg he had developed an ulcer. Unhealed, it was the reason for his swollen ankle. Operation to remove his varicosities and local treatment of his leg ulcer soon removed both the leg swelling and anxiety about his heart.

Many cardiophobes forget about their heart in cool

166

weather and begin to worry all over again every summer when a heat spell brings on ankle swelling. If you are overweight and have a job which requires standing most of the day, it is not unlikely that you may have some leg swelling. I have noted this often in women who stand behind the counters of department stores. Although the air conditioning keeps the heat factor down, the lack of movement pools the blood in the leg veins and is conducive to leg swelling.

I recall a young woman who broke her leg while skiing. It was a bad break and the limb was in a cast for many weeks. After the cast was removed, she had the ankle and leg swelling which is not uncommon in such circumstances. She accepted this without anxiety. But when the swelling lasted for several months, she became frightened.

"For the first time in my life I became introspective," she told me. "I could only explain the puffiness as a symptom that my heart was beginning to weaken. My family doctor kept reassuring me that my heart was all right, but I didn't regain confidence in it until all the swelling had disappeared for good."

If you have unexplained ankle swelling, and if the possibility of heart disease sneaks into your consciousness, then you should hasten to your doctor for two reasons: 1. To get a head start *forgetting* about it if the verdict turns out to be imaginary heart trouble. 2. To get a head start *treating* it—if you really do have heart disease.

11.

FATIGUE? THE HEART IS OFTEN INNOCENT

Fatigue is a common symptom of heart disease, but it is a more common complaint in people with healthy hearts. Few of those who come to doctors with complaints about fatigue suffer from cardiac disability. They suffer dis-ease but not disease.

If you are always tired, what I have said should encourage you. Fatigue can be deadening, of course. It blunts the edge of living. But it need not be the bugaboo it has become with some individuals.

One day four women were sitting around a bridge table, munching cookies and sipping tea after having played a few rubbers of bridge. I had just left the husband of the hostess in another part of the house. He was in bed with a bad back. His orthopedist had him in traction. Since he was a personal friend as well as a patient, I had dropped by to say hello.

As I edged toward the front door to leave, the hostess of the bridge game waved me over to have a few cookies and tea. Since three of the women were patients and old friends, I could not beg off. Later, I was glad I accepted her invitation because the conversation soon turned to the problems of the fourth woman—a house guest from another city.

My three patients had been acting as amateur medical advisers for this lady. Like most gratuitous advice, theirs had not been well received. Nevertheless, what they had told her made good sense.

It appears that the lady had been complaining that she suffered from extreme fatigue as well as daily doubt about her heart's performance. Because my three patients had lately been through similar prolonged sieges of fatigue, each had her own special brand of advice to offer the out-of-town guest.

The hostess asked me to sit down after she had introduced me. She said, "Helen, why don't you tell our doctor what you have told us about yourself? Since this is Sunday and he can't escape us, he will just have to listen—and perhaps offer you some good advice."

The visitor was a concerned, frail-looking woman of about forty-five. At first, she remonstrated against the imposition of my being asked professional advice on "my day off." But on the insistence of the hostess and myself, she began:

"Doctor, I suppose you hear this complaint in your office every day: fatigue. I'm just beat. Too tired to go to sleep at night. Too tired to get out of bed in the morning. I've given up all civic work. No more committees. No more concerts or theater. I have to push myself to go to an occasional movie. My two children are married. Fortunately, they left home to be married when I was still myself. But my husband is the one who is catching it. One day I'm sure he will leave in disgust.

"I haven't told him—and I've kept it from the girls here, until now—what really is on my mind. This constant exhaustion has become so intensified that I've been worrying about my heart. This is my big worry. More than the tiredness.

"My doctor says *no,* but I say *yes,* I *do* have a weak heart. I've been taking tonics and tranquilizers. Nothing helps. I appreciate the advice your three patients have been offering me, but I'm afraid I'm too far gone to hope for any help."

She looked at me, raised her eyebrows questioningly, as if to say, "There's the entire, hopeless story in a nutshell"—and slumped back in her chair, her gray eyes somehow emphasizing the weariness that suffused her body.

I turned to my three patients. "You say each one of you has given your friend some advice. As your doctor-teacher, I'm interested in your suggestions."

Our hostess was first. "You remember, doctor, what a mess I was when I first came to you. I was tired all the time, heart palpitating, certain that I was about to die any minute. For a month I had been taking vitamins, trying to build myself up. I had been too scared to come in for an examination and hear the true diagnosis. Suppose it's really heart disease, I kept asking myself. But Jack [her husband] finally brought me in.

"At first I didn't believe it when you said my heart was all right. The fatigue was still overpowering me. Not until you discovered that I had a lazy thyroid, did I begin to improve by taking three grains of thyroid extract every day.

"Now I feel like a new woman. This is what I told Helen: Get your doctor to check up on your thyroid gland."

I turned to patient number two on my right. "Now it's

171

your turn," I said. "Let's see what you've learned by being a patient of mine. What advice did you give?"

She said, "I know what tiredness to the point of exhaustion means. I know the terrible fears that go with loss of confidence in your heart. Exhaustion and heart fear was the two-headed monster that tormented me from day to day.

"I've told Helen she can't possibly feel any worse than I did. Always nervous, trembly, and afraid. Who wouldn't feel that way with a heart skipping all over the chest? I told her what my trouble was. That little nodule in my thyroid gland was doing the opposite of our hostess'. My gland was too active instead of being too lazy.

"Hyperthyroidism had been making a mess of me. An operation took care of it. I'm a new woman now, too. The way I play golf and tennis and cavort around the dance floor for hours has certainly convinced me that I must have a heart as strong as anyone's."

The third friend then chimed in: "All I told her was to have her doctor check her blood sugar. As in my case, hypoglycemia may be the reason for her exhaustion and heart fears. My low blood sugar, as you know, was soon brought under control by a high-protein diet and by staying away from sweets. It's made me what I am today —a heart-happy, grateful woman."

I studied all the ladies gathered around me, assessing their opinions against what I had heard from Helen, before I replied.

"Frankly," I told them, "there is merit in all the advice you ladies have offered to Helen. Each of the causative factors mentioned could be responsible for her difficulties. However, don't rule out involutional melancholia."

"What is that?" Helen inquired, her curiosity piqued.

"It involves a lessening of ovarian activity that usually

occurs as women approach middle age and go into menopause. Very often this combination of factors brings on a kind of involuntary depression. On the surface there seems to be no cause for the melancholia, yet invariably it is connected with the lessened activity I have mentioned."

My tentative diagnosis started a round of animated talking among the ladies. However, since I had a busy day ahead of me, I excused myself and hurried on home.

What happened to Helen? I heard later from my hostess that a further complete study made by her physician turned up negative findings except for one diagnosis—involutional melancholia. She was having an unusually hard time in her menopause. In fact, she had confessed this fact to the hostess and the other ladies after my departure.

Because energizers, tranquilizers, and hormones hadn't helped, she was given a course of electric-sleep therapy. She, too, improved. About six months later, I saw the four of them around a bridge table again. I dubbed them, in my own mind, "the happy foursome."

What I have been saying is that there are many causes of fatigue that can produce apprehension about one's heart. It is the job of both the patient and the doctor to try to ferret out any hidden and deep conflicts that can result in chronic anxiety. This is not invariably easy. It takes time, money, and patience. If the family doctor cannot provide it, perhaps the psychiatrist can.

One day I received the following note from a concerned wife:

My husband is an industrialist. I wish he were just an ordinary, relaxed working man, like he used to be years ago. I've found luxury but lost the companionship of a husband. I wish for the good old days, although I am too young to have known them firsthand, when men were relaxed and took their time eating, when they didn't work like ants busy rebuilding. Modern businessmen aren't as sensible as their grandfathers.

Here is my reply:

Whenever I hear anyone mention the good old days, I know he or she is letting imagination run away with him. Human nature hasn't changed much in a few generations.

Let me tell you about the good old days. I have been reading an interesting book by William Blaikie, published in 1879 and called *How to Get Strong.* I don't agree with all he says about exercise, but I think you too will be interested in his statements about businessmen. Remember, however, that he is writing about men working in the nineteenth century:

"Who does not know about his friends, businessmen whose faces show they are nearly all the time overworked; who get thin, and stay so; who look tired and are so; who go dragging along throughout their duties. . . . The noon meal is rushed through, perhaps when the brain is at white-heat. More is eaten, both then and in the evening than they will digest—then comes broken sleep. The man waking from it is not rested, is not rebuilt and strong, and ready for the new day. What wonder is it that nervous exhaustion is so frequent among them."

Then he quotes from *Wear and Tear,* a book written by the famous Dr. S. Weir Mitchell, who was a specialist in diseases of the nervous system:

". . . I have met with numerous instances of nervous exhaustion among merchants and manufacturers. My notebooks seem to show that manufacturers and

174

certain classes of railway officials are the most liable to suffer from neural exhaustion. Next to these come merchants in general, brokers, etc.; then, less frequently, clergymen; still less often lawyers; and, more rarely, doctors; while distressing cases are apt to occur among the overschooled young of both sexes."

There were overworked businessmen in the good old days, too. It is not so much the era as it is the nature of the man (or woman) that counts.

Tension is the common enemy. It is the opposite of relaxation. Imaginary heart trouble feeds on it and is fed by it. Tension has a ravenous appetite. It weakens man's reserves so that he lives in fatigue. And when he is exhausted day after day, he is like a ripe tomato ready to be sliced by a sharp knife; exhaustion peels off the layers of energy until there is nothing left but fear.

Fear of the heart, of the lungs, of the stomach—every organ in the body is a potential target for the exhausted. Men and women should realize this.

Unfortunately, many look straight into the face of the problem of fatigue and the effect it has on the normal heart, as if it were of no consequence.

For example, I recall one woman who did not understand the simple demands of a tired husband. He complained of palpitation and heart pains, and she called him a hypochondriac before their friends. Being physically active herself (a champion tennis player and an enthusiastic jogger) she wanted her husband to become more active.

One day she complained to me, "My husband is too lazy. He is only twenty-eight and it bothers me to see him lying around on weekends. He acts as if he were sixty-five as soon as Saturday arrives. He likes to stretch out in a hammock, either reading or daydreaming. It's all I can do to get him to mow the lawn or fix a few

175

things around the house. Only occasionally does he go out to play golf.

"He keeps telling me he gets enough exercise on the job all week. He says, 'I work hard in my job as a letter carrier. I walk miles. When the weekend comes, I just want to take it easy. It's my way of recharging my battery. What's wrong with that?' Doctor, this is about our only bone of contention. What does one do with a lazy husband?"

I agreed that a married man has certain responsibilities to his family on weekends, as well as on any other day.

"It is certainly his job, not yours to mow the lawn and do necessary house repairs," I told her. "And if your kids want to go out on a picnic, dad should gladly volunteer, no matter how much he'd prefer to lie around. He is twenty-eight and old enough to know that when you're married you can't be as carefree as a beachcomber.

"But there's another side to it. Remember, when he is stretched out in lazy comfort, that each of us is different and responds to his own needs. For example, what type of body build does your husband conform to? Is he a mesomorph or ectomorph? [Medium built or thin and wiry?] Or, is he an endomorph? [Not so much muscular as weighty with excess fat?]

"If he is endomorphic, he is naturally lazy physically. That alone is reason enough for his wanting to avoid activity on weekends. But even if he fits into the muscular and active classifications, he may still prefer to take it easy because he is tired from the effort spent in working during the week.

"It's an old, tired simile, but when he says, 'It's my way of recharging my battery,' it comes as close to describing it as anything else. Since he has also been com-

176

plaining of palpitation and heart pains, I wouldn't push him into doing anything that doesn't come naturally. Otherwise fatigue will increase and his imaginary heart trouble will also loom more importantly in his mind.

"Let him play golf if he wishes, or just rest if he'd rather relax. He says he gets his full exercise during the week, so there is no deficiency there.

"Of course, it's possible that your husband is too lazy, as you say, but it's also possible that you are unnecessarily goading him on. If too much unnatural activity on the weekend only serves to exhaust him, then he will surely become inefficient and unhappy on his job, and spend the rest of the time worrying about his heart."

As in everything else, I told her, it's better to live and let live. Otherwise, I warned, she ran the risk of having a very unhappy man on her hands for the rest of her life. Once her husband lost complete confidence in his heart, he might turn into a semi-invalid at work and at home. In that case, she might be sorry she didn't allow him to fall into his natural niche of physical laziness.

I have known many men who began to doubt the efficiency of their heart because they were "always tired." Questioning elicited the information that exhaustion was due to overwork and inability to relax on weekends. As I've said elsewhere, moonlighting is another way of inviting imaginary heart trouble. Fatigue is the breeding ground for symptoms that incorrectly convict the heart.

A common type of imaginary heart trouble is effort syndrome. It was also called soldier's heart because so many tired, nervous young men suffer from it while in the military service. They become as incapacitated as if they had real heart disease.

In this condition extensive tests reveal no organic change

177

in the heart or in the rest of the body to account for the patient's symptoms. He is at the mercy of any slight exertion that tires him.

These patients cannot put in a full day's work—at school or in a job. After a few hours they are exhausted. They complain of indigestion, chest pain, heart skips, palpitation, low spirits—but mostly of exhaustion. Fatigue is the daily cross they bear. Too tired to eat or sleep, they force themselves to get through the morning (if they can), but crumble in spirit and physical ability by midafternoon.

Often the sympathetic family doctor can help, but the psychiatrist must not be forgotten as the last court of appeal in stubborn cases of effort syndrome.

If you can face up to yourself honestly as being a cardiophobe, then ask yourself the reason for your chronic tiredness and debility. If you can answer without prodding or prompting, you will certainly not need the services of any physician—family doctor or psychiatrist.

Do you hate your job? Here is an overlooked, common reason for chronic fatigue! You can't get up morning after morning, with such unpleasant feelings tearing you apart, without at last surrendering to exhaustion—and to the long train of symptoms that usually follow. Change your work (not easy, I know) and you may cure yourself overnight. Palpitations, skips, pains, and other alarming symptoms will disappear.

Do you hate the person who works beside you? Do you dislike your mother-in-law? Your wife? Your husband? Your children? Admit it—although it takes courage—and you are on your way to a cure. Do you resent someone who has made more money than you have; or who got the job promotion you expected to be your own? Forget it if you can, and you may become a healthy man overnight.

178

Are you weary because you live in indecision? Can't you even pick out a necktie without going through the formality of making an earth-shattering decision? Learn to be more decisive, and much fatigue will disappear.

Emotional conflict can also cause fatigue. Someone has likened it to an automobile running with its brakes on—a reason why neurotics expend so much energy.

Maybe you're always tired because you have been starving yourself. In this land of plenty, many (through carelessness or inability to purchase food) get insufficient nourishment. Are you vitamin-starved, too?

Such are some of the apparently unimportant reasons for fatigue that wears away your reserves as surely as ocean waves wear away the sands of a beach.

I asked two former world-champion boxers how they overcome anxiety. The weeks of training before a fight would be useless for efficiency in the ring if fatigue took over and sapped their physical strength.

How do they exist during those months of the training grind before a fight? What kept them in one piece?

I asked these questions of Floyd Patterson in a personal interview while he was preparing for his second fight with Ingemar Johansson, the man who had knocked him out and taken his title away from him.

A gentle, quiet man outside the ring, Patterson answered simply and frankly, "I have no room for fear. I do not think of it; not that I am trying to run away from it. And I am not trying to build up my confidence by talking this way; it is a part of me. My days and nights are taken up with preparing my body so that it will be in top physical condition on the day of the fight. I think only of winning; never of the possibility of losing. I do my job, live day by day, and have faith. I guess you can call it positive thinking as much as anything else. I don't

179

allow myself to think negative. If you want the secret that may help your patients, perhaps it's in that last sentence. *Don't think negative*."

Not bad reasoning when you consider that he regained his title.

A few days later I met another gentleman outside the ring, one of our greatest boxing champions. Joe Louis was walking across a hotel lobby when I stopped to ask him the same questions. (Having been in the ring as an amateur for only two rounds during my entire lifetime, I nevertheless feel an instinctive association with, and respect for, boxers because in those few minutes I had learned the meaning of fear. And I knew the anxiety I had suffered for a few days before my own bout.)

I introduced myself and said, "How do you train for a fight? Not your muscles, but your mind—so you won't be scared."

Like Patterson, he considered the questions for a moment, then replied, "I was so busy getting ready, there was no time for fear. I was always confident—not in any boastful way—that I would win. My manager used to say to me, 'Just fight one round at a time, Joe.' Then the next one, and the one after that. Until I won. In that way, there's no time for fear. One thing at a time. People who think too far ahead can get themselves into a tizzy. That's the secret. When you think only of winning, nothing can scare you. Too many people think of losing—and that makes them scared of life."

Since those interviews I have told frightened and anxious people to think of winning their health rather than losing it. It's not easy, but neither do champions find it easy to live from day to day.

If you have been losing the battle of exhaustion, if your

heart has been cutting the customary capers tired people experience, if you are tempted to surrender to fear and imaginary heart trouble, then you might be one of the fortunate ones who decide to put up a fight—like the champions did. Leave no room for anxiety.

Look at yourself honestly—a full-length view in the mirror, as honestly close to your thoughts and beliefs as you can get without the immediate help of a doctor. There are many questions that you must ask yourself and answer.

They are inherent in the following thoughts by R. V. C. Bodley in his *In Search of Serenity,* as described by A. Powell Davis:

> The chief barriers to serenity, especially in America, Mr. Bodley sees as worry over self-importance and social standing, worry over financial problems and work, worry brought about by physical indulgence, worry attendant upon love and marriage, worry about politics and world affairs, and finally worry about death.

A good exercise in overcoming unnecessary anxiety is checking off these items one by one. Think of all the questions they stir up inside yourself—provided, as I said, you are completely honest with yourself.

Is your social standing so important to you? Must you live up to the Joneses or find yourself unhappy? Are you bored and frustrated sitting in the back row instead of being one of the important men on the dais? Does your work worry you? Why? Are you richer than you think? Do you overburden your physical body with too much alcohol, tobacco, work? Is your marriage a source of your unhappiness and anxiety? What are you doing about it?

Fatigue is the common enemy. In the susceptible it

181

breeds chronic anxiety. In the especially susceptible it breeds heart fear. Is the fatigue due to a faulty way of living? Then relief depends upon yourself.

One way or another, with your cooperation and with your doctor's dedicated help, you can wipe out—or learn to live with—many, or all, of the symptoms that have made you lose faith in your heart's capacity to keep you alive and well.

12.

IS YOUR HEART TROUBLE
REAL OR IMAGINARY?
(A Summary)

Do you have heart symptoms? Better ask yourself (and your doctor) again if your heart trouble is real or imaginary. Not only your happiness, but your life often depends upon the correct answer.

It is likely that at some time in your life you have had heart trouble—the Romeo-Juliet type of affliction. For most of us, the sweet, throbbing beats of the heart-in-love are welcome.

Not so with real heart symptoms. We spread no welcome mat for them. Nobody who is in love with life can minimize their implications and threats.

Anxiety about one's heart is inevitable in a country in which at least 10,000,000 people have organic (real) cardiovascular disease; and in which at least 15,000,000 additional frustrated and disheartened persons *think* they have heart disease but actually do not. Directly or indirectly, the heart problem affects each of us. Therefore, we—doctors and patients—should put our heads together to overcome heart trouble—whether it be real or imaginary.

Joshua Loth Liebman has written:

Yet it is correct to maintain that all human beings without exception—or with the exception of the moron or idiot—experience fear and worry.

Recently I saw two patients who illustrate the divergent reactions to heart awareness that doctors observe routinely.

One was a successful lawyer of fifty who said, "Doctor, I really don't see why I can't play thirty-six holes of golf on weekends. I know I had a coronary occlusion six months ago, but I've taken it easy until now. I'd rather not play at all than only be allowed to play only nine holes a day."

The other was a forty-five-year-old owner and manager of a small electronics firm. "Doctor," he said, "I wish I could believe you, but I can't get it out of my mind that one of these days I'm going to drop in my tracks. When it begins to skip all over the place it's hard to believe that my heart is all right."

Here, in miniature, you have observed one man with a bad heart who disregards the red light, and another with a perfectly normal heart who doesn't dare drive through the green light. In his daily living routine, one refuses to use the brake, the other the accelerator.

If your heart trouble is real, it is senseless to minimize it. If it is imaginary, take steps to neutralize your discomforts.

To overcome needless heart worry, visit your doctor for a complete cardiac evaluation. Remember that the stethoscope is not sufficient for modern heart diagnosis. You will need the diagnostic works: complete physical examination; fluoroscopic, X-ray and electrocardiographic studies, and laboratory examinations.

Modern doctors don't pat you on the back reassuringly

184

if your heart is not up to par. They don't say, "Forget it"; they tell you the truth—and what to do about it, depending upon what kind of involvement you have.

Therefore, if your doctor says, "Your heart is normal" —believe him and be thankful you are all right. Banish your previous doubts. Many persons do so on hearing the good news; others continue to be apprehensive in spite of the doctor's verdict of "not guilty."

Why, then, are so many millions of Americans unnecessarily heart-conscious? There are many reasons:

Perhaps you were recently turned down for insurance because of an inconsequential murmur or border-line blood pressure.

Perhaps you have become upset by the death of a close friend who had been suffering from heart trouble.

Is it possible that you are unduly aware of your heart because you have for months nursed a member of your family incapacitated by heart disease?

Perhaps you have grown up from childhood as a "heart invalid"; you were kept away from gym and active sports because of a negligible heart murmur.

There are other causes of imaginary heart trouble: *heart symptoms*. Having one or more of them may transform you into a heart-worrier: Palpitation, heart skips, pain in the left chest, pain in the left shoulder or arm, shortness of breath, swelling of the ankles, tiredness, cough, and indigestion are the usual scaremongers.

Therefore, remember this: *You may have one or all of the aforementioned symptoms, yet not have heart disease!*

Palpitation and heart skips may be found in the healthiest of hearts. Pain in the left chest is rarely due to heart disease; it is usually the result of nerve or muscle inflammation. Shortness of breath may be caused by overweight

185

or being unused to exertion. Swelling of the ankles may be the effect of excessive heat and protracted walking or standing. Tiredness, due to lack of rest; cough, due to too much smoking, and indigestion due to a rebellious stomach, complete the picture.

If you are overworked, sleepless, and overtired; if daily exhaustion has added up to chronic fatigue; if you are nervous due to an underlying anxiety—then you are a candidate for imaginary heart trouble. Do something about it.

Don't guess. Have your doctor differentiate between the real and the unreal. Don't hesitate to find out. *Maybe it isn't your heart!*

"I was sure my heart was going to jump right out yesterday," said a housewife. "It began to beat fast and race —like a frightened bird trying to get away."

Examination revealed a normal heart. Her symptoms were due to emotional imbalance.

A forty-five-year-old lumberyard operator said to me recently, "I've had this pain over my left chest for the past three days. I have a suspicion my heart must be getting weak."

Questioning revealed that he had become frightened about himself after hearing of the death of a friend. Electrocardiographic and other studies proved his heart was normal.

These are only two specific instances of the hundreds of ways in which imaginary heart sufferers complain of their symptoms.

Most of these people are over thirty-five. (As a rule, youngsters are not so unduly aware of their physical condition.) As people reach the shady side of forty naturally they become more concerned about their health. Symptoms begin to plague the more sensitive and susceptible individuals.

Does your heart seem, at times, to run away like a frightened colt? Does it hop, skip, and jump? Do you have sticking, achy pains in your left chest? Do you have a premonition that your days are numbered? You, too, may have symptoms of heart disease, yet have a normal heart, just like those people who complain of palpitation, shortness of breath, ankle swelling, indigestion, tiredness, cough, or heart skips.

A recent divorcee said, "I thought I'd die last night. My heart began skipping when I got into bed. After each skip it seemed like an eternity before the next beat would come along. I was sure each beat was my last."

Her heart, although irritable because of emotional stress and tension, was normal.

In the same way, indigestion—sometimes a symptom of heart trouble—may be due to something not connected with the heart. For example, it may be caused by a faulty gall bladder.

Tiredness may be due to overwork—mental or physical, or it may be due to a slight deficiency in iron in the blood or to an underactive thyroid, or to various conditions unrelated to the heart.

Shortness of breath may be caused by a physiological slowing up. Many of us after forty just can't get used to climbing a flight or two of stairs. Excess weight may do it, too.

Without question, some of the worst sufferers from "heart trouble" are those who don't have heart disease. *They just have the symptoms.* And they are the ones who die a thousand deaths because they are too frightened to learn the truth.

It must be understood, of course, that I am not eliminating the possibility that certain individuals who display one or more of the symptoms we have mentioned may actually have organic heart disease. Chest pain *may* be due to coronary occlusion; ankle swelling, tiredness, shortness of breath *may* be due to a failing heart.

But why *guess* when the odds are in your favor that your heart is doing a good job? Think of all the fun you miss, all the activities you unnecessarily curtail, because you *guess* that your heart is not up to par. I have known hundreds of patients who have given up golf, gardening, bowling, long walks simply because they had a symptom or two; yet, they were blessed with normal hearts.

The proper course of action is to see your doctor if you are unduly anxious about your heart. If he says it's doing fine, I assure you that finding a million dollars in your pocket won't make you feel so elated (for a while, at least!).

But suppose he says: "Your heart's all right except that it's beginning to show some signs of wear. Nothing serious. Just a matter of following my advice and it will be on the job until you're seventy or eighty."

There's nothing too bad with a verdict like that either.

The answer to this whole problem of heart trouble seems to be obvious. If you have heart symptoms, find out if the trouble is *imaginary* or *real*.

In other words, it is better to stop *guessing* about your heart and start *knowing*. To paraphrase the old saying: "Doctor knows best." Leave it up to him.

PART III

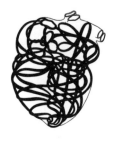

SPECIFIC ADVICE
FOR THE HEART-SICK

13.

YOUR BLOOD PRESSURE

"Why borrow trouble?" This is one of the most common reasons people give for not going to the doctor while they are well. More than the time loss and money spent, I think the fear that the doctor will find something they don't suspect (because they've felt well) is the motivating reason for their procrastination.

The other day a friend of mine remarked to me, "I've been feeling perfect. Although I'm forty-eight, I've never had a physical. Why should I? I'd only be borrowing trouble. There's time enough for going to doctors when illness strikes."

Not always. For example, consider high blood pressure. It is important because it is one of the most commonly associated conditions with coronary heart disease. If you have high blood pressure for ten years, you increase at least four times the risk of getting a heart attack. If, in addition, you are overweight, have diabetes and a high cholesterol content in your blood, the chances of having coronary thrombosis are many times greater.

For this reason alone, it is important to have a checkup even though you are feeling well. Actually, you may experience no adverse reactions despite the fact that your pressure is abnormally high.

I'll never forget a woman in her sixties who came in to see me a number of years ago because she was concerned about a small growth on her chin. During the examination, I discovered that her blood pressure was over 250. It taught me a lesson: patients with such high pressures often feel well. They may have no history of headaches, dizziness, or shortness of breath.

Yet, they may be in danger because of the prolonged effect of high blood pressure on the heart and coronary blood vessels, and on the vessels of the brain and kidneys.

Sometimes a patient will visit his eye specialist to be fitted for new lenses. Feeling apparently well, he is greatly chagrined when told that there are signs in the back of his eyes (during ophthalmoscopic examination) that indicate trouble with his arteries. On going to his family doctor or to an internist he learns, for the first time, that he has abnormally high blood pressure. With the newer drugs now available to control high blood pressure, it is too bad that so many still say, "Why borrow trouble?"

A housewife recently said to me, "I have been plagued by severe headaches lately. About a year ago I was told that my blood pressure is high. To tell you the truth, I'm afraid to return to the doctor. Most likely, he'll say that my blood pressure is way up."

If you are an apparently healthy person, you will probably attribute a headache to tension. If you have high blood pressure, however, you are likely to say, "My headache's worse because my pressure must be sky-high today." But there is not much scientific evidence to support the theory that headaches are caused by a blood-pressure rise.

Dr. I. M. G. Stewart wrote in the British medical periodical *Lancet* of his studies of this symptom in a large number of cases. He concluded that so-called hypertension headache is, in reality, an anxiety and tension symptom.

He studied 200 patients with high blood pressure and only one in four complained of headaches. He mentioned 104 patients who did not know they had hypertension, and 87 denied having headaches.

In another paper written for the *Journal of the American Medical Association,* Drs. M. Moser, H. Wish, and A. P. Friedman found that 43 of 54 patients definitely complained of headaches from one to 25 years *before* the high blood pressure began.

You might expect, with the use of the very efficient blood-pressure-lowering drugs that headaches would disappear. But such has not been the case. Only 25 percent of patients so treated experienced definite relief from headache when the pressure was lowered.

Therefore, I suggest again, that persons with high blood pressure should not go to pieces emotionally if they suffer severe headaches. The symptom doesn't invariably signify that your pressure is taking off like a missile. You may discover, if you look hard enough, that the cause is some unpleasant environmental factor at home or at work. If you cannot find the reason, it makes good sense to turn the responsibility over to your doctor.

In spite of many recent advances in treatment by the new wonder drugs (we don't hear much these days about operative treatment like "sympathectomies") too many patients with high blood pressure live in frustration and fear. When the column of mercury climbs in the blood-pressure machine, they break up.

"What's the pressure today, Doctor?" they ask fearfully.

You don't have time to remove the stethoscope from your ears. Their frightened eyes look into yours as they wait for the "bad news."

For the purpose of bringing such people solace and hope, I am reprinting a letter which I received several months ago:

> I am writing to you in regard to a letter I read in your column. It was written by Mrs. T. She stated her ailments as high blood pressure, dropsy and poor vision. Her age was fifty-six. I know she will be interested to know that I had somewhat similar trouble at the age of forty-two. I was in bed for almost a year and grew worse as the days went by.
>
> Our family doctor said he could only give me shots to reduce the fluid in my body. I had a very bad spell one night. The next morning a specialist was called who put me in the hospital. The doctor said I would have lived only two weeks at the most if the new wonder drugs did not work—with God to help.
>
> My blood pressure was way over 200 and my pump was stretched. When I was admitted, the actual figures of my pressure were 280 over 140. Any doctor will tell you how apparently hopeless such a pressure is.
>
> When I entered the hospital, I weighed 190 pounds. When I was discharged fifty days later, I weighed 119 pounds. I had to buy a blood pressure cuff and learn to take my own pressure. My blood pressure now stays between 130 and 145. My heart is smaller and stronger. Of course, I make visits to the doctor's office to be checked and have my medicines regulated.
>
> There is now no swelling in my optic nerves at all. The doctors are proud of my case.
>
> I thought this letter might give some of your readers a lift. Especially those who worry so much about a few-point rise in blood pressure. When they think of

me they will stop worrying so much. Please also mention that I am not an invalid. I am able to be up, cook, dust, go to the movies, ride, walk, climb stairs, plant flowers, and go to church.

There you have it in its entirety—a message from one kindly soul to all of you who "need a lift."

This patient's history is revealing. It gives evidence of her faith that she would eventually recover (which is so important, whatever the illness). It also serves as a practical example of how a heart overburdened by having to pump against an abnormally high pressure shows its relief from strain after the pressure has been brought down to normal limits.

Controlling high blood pressure is as important in preventing heart disease as in treating it. The heart cannot perform an adequate job when it is laboring against a high pressure.

14.

LOW BLOOD PRESSURE

There is an old saying "Leave well enough alone" which applies especially to patients who have low blood pressure. Until lately, both doctors and patients were in the habit of tinkering with good machines simply because the pressure was "lower than normal." At last, doctors have come to realize that low blood pressure is an asset rather than a liability.

Nevertheless, too many laymen still believe that something ought to be done about their low blood pressure. Not a week goes by in which most doctors do not see patients who want their blood pressure brought up to "normal."

"Doctor," a patient will say, "I had an insurance examination last month. They found my pressure was on the low side. Don't you think I ought to do something about it?"

The doctor answers the question with a question: "Did you get the policy?"

If the answer is yes, the patient has his answer. Insurance company statistics have shown that when your blood pressure is on the low side, your expected life is at least as long as (usually longer than) that of your neighbor who has normal pressure.

Of course, there are a few conditions in medicine in which a chronic, low pressure is associated with abnormality. For example, in Addison's disease, pressures may be much below 100. In this condition, however, there are other specific symptoms and signs that influence the diagnosis: pigmentation of the skin, extreme weakness, and disturbance in the body's salt metabolism.

Suppose, however, that you are feeling well and that a routine examination indicates your systolic blood pressure is 90 or 100. That's nothing to be alarmed about. I have seen systolic pressures of 90 and 100 in big, strapping athletes.

I am sure your doctor will tell you that you are fortunate to have a low blood pressure in this high-pressure world we are living in today. Do not expect him to give you shots or iron or vitamin capsules to bring your pressure back to normal. Be thankful it is on the low side rather than climbing.

In 95 percent of the cases, we don't know what causes high blood pressure. The same percentage holds true for pressures on the low side. That being so, it is better not to tinker.

Of course, there are times when patients with low blood pressure complain of easy fatigue, loss of energy, and a tendency to be drowsy during the day. Such patients should be investigated for the underlying cause of such symptoms. It is easy, but often wrong, to attribute them to low blood pressure.

For example, your doctor may discover that you have low blood pressure *plus* secondary anemia. A course of iron tablets will benefit the anemia and restore your energy. Nevertheless, your blood pressure may remain low

—which is all right. Likewise, your symptoms may be due to a mild hypothyroid state. If your basal metabolism is low, a few thyroid tablets daily as prescribed by your doctor will transform your lethargy into pep.

In other words, be thankful for low blood pressure. Don't use it as a scapegoat when you have symptoms. Look for other causes of your discomfort.

Many people continue to be perturbed instead of thankful for a pressure on the low side. I know that many take injections, tonics, and other treatments to raise it. They are wasting time and money. I never prescribe medicines to raise it, as there isn't any medicine that will keep pressure higher indefinitely. Low blood pressure should not be a problem for patients unless it is quite low as a result of underlying disease.

If you are concerned about your heart because you suffer from dizziness, fatigue, faintness, or shortness of breath, I realize there is a measure of relief in thinking you have found the culprit: low blood pressure. But all this kind of thinking does is add another notch to the belt of anxiety—unnecessarily. Whereas ordinary high blood pressure may be hurtful if not treated, ordinary low blood pressure is harmless—whether you treat it or not.

15.

RHEUMATIC
HEART DISEASE

Brevity may be the soul of wit, but it certainly taxes the will power of the writer who often must condense a volume of information into a few hundred words. Where to begin? How much to say? Where to end? Well, let's begin.

Rheumatic heart disease is not caused, as many think, by rheumatism. It is true that the infection in the heart precipitated by the streptococcus germ may precede inflammation of the joints or follow such painful swellings. However, they happen to be different manifestations of the same process. Most cases of rheumatic heart disease begin in childhood and in the teens. Here is a typical case history:

Jimmy, age fourteen, stays home from school for a few days because he has a painful sore throat and fever. He returns to school, apparently fully recovered. A few weeks later he begins to complain of painful, swollen knees or wrists or ankles. He has a fever.

For the first time, a doctor is called. He makes the diagnosis of rheumatic fever. It is at this stage that the doctor is especially careful to determine if there are any heart complications. For he knows that the joints, as I have said, are only one facet of the problem. And he knows that not all patients get heart involvement.

But as he listens to Jimmy's heart he hears a tell-tale murmur indicating that a heart valve (as well as heart muscle) has been attacked by the bacteria. For this reason he advises that Jimmy have complete rest in bed for weeks (sometimes for months). The purpose is to lessen heart damage. The doctor also prescribes antibiotics, aspirin, and cortisone drugs to lessen infection.

In order to try to prevent further attacks of a similar nature that might further damage the heart, the doctor prescribes sulfa drugs or penicillin which Jimmy will take for months and years to set up this wall of defense.

What is the best way to prevent future attacks? By giving pills or injections? One doctor prescribes pills to be taken every day, while another believes in giving an injection once a month. In a recent issue of the *Journal of the American Medical Association,* there is an instructive article on this point—"Prophylaxis of Recurrent Rheumatic Fever," written by Dr. Alvan R. Feinstein of New Haven and five associates.

They observed 343 young rheumatic patients during four calendar years, Here are a few of their findings:

> It now seems clear that neither oral sulfadiazine nor any of the oral penicillin prophylactic regimens we have tested has the antirheumatic effectiveness of a single monthly injection of penicillin G benzathine—none of the simple oral regimens equals the effectiveness of long-lasting injectable penicillin G benzathine in the prevention of rheumatic fever.
>
> Thus, the injections are clearly the preparation of choice when the most effective form of antirheumatic

202

prophylaxis is desired. In rheumatic patients who have no or minimal heart disease, however, rheumatic recurrences carry little risk of cardiac damage. An oral preparation [pill] for such patients is acceptable, and may be desirable to avoid the disadvantages of monthly injections.

So it is evident that there is something to say both for the doctor who advises penicillin or sulfadiazine by mouth, and the one who recommends monthly injections of penicillin. Much will depend upon classification into which the patient fits.

Not all patients who have rheumatic fever get heart involvement. But suppose one does? What happens to the heart?

You have heard that the heart is a pump. Well, like many efficient pumps, it has valves. Normally, these fit tightly when they close, and the heart pumps efficiently. However, after serious injury by the streptococcus, scars form and these valves produce a leakage.

You know how hard you have to pump water with a leaky pump. That happens when a heart has leaky valves due to rheumatic infection. (Not, I repeat, when there are harmless functional murmurs.) As a result of the extra effort over many years, the heart muscle gets larger and larger to compensate for the valve injury. Finally the time arrives when it can no longer do the job well with leaky valves and the patient has what we call heart failure—with the symptoms of shortness of breath, swollen ankles, cough, weakness, dizziness, among others.

In short, that's just about what rheumatic heart disease is. Warning: If your child complains of sore throat and fever, don't treat him with home remedies. If the sore throat lasts longer than a day or two, have your doctor make a throat swab, and send it to the laboratory. If the infection is due to the streptococcus germ, only penicillin, other antibiotics, and the sulfa drugs will hold it in check. The best way to treat it and the best way to prevent it is always to be suspicious of your child's sore throat. With or without inflammation of the joints, it is possible that the heart may be involved.

Whenever in doubt as to whether a child has suffered heart damage, it is advisable to request the pediatrician or family doctor to invite the opinion of a heart specialist. Laboratory examinations and special electrocardiograms may be necessary in making the correct diagnosis, especially in doubtful cases.

Rheumatic heart disease is not the enigma it was a few years ago. We can control it better with antibiotics and other heart medications. Even when these fail we can fall back on cardiac surgery and substitute plastic valves for damaged heart valves. I have known apparently hopeless rheumatic cardiacs who lived for many years after such restorative operations.

People should remember that rheumatic fever does not affect everyone in the same way. At least 50 percent of patients come through without even getting a heart complication. And most of those who have actual heart disease may live out normal lives. Others, depending upon the amount of involvement in the valves and heart muscle, may have to curtail some activities.

Many women with rheumatic heart disease begin to worry about their first pregnancy. Can they have a baby? This is uppermost in their mind. Such patients have had more than one child without difficulty.

I recall sitting next to an attractive young social worker at a party given by one of my patients. Because I was introduced to her as a doctor, she said, "I think you'll be interested in my medical history. I had rheumatic fever

204

when I was about seven years old and was left with a heart murmur which my doctor said is due to rheumatic heart disease. Although I am only thirty I am the mother of six children—twelve, ten, eight, six, four and two.

"So far my heart has never bothered me. Yet, when I was a child I wasn't allowed to climb stairs and take part in any strenuous activities. But I got married at sixteen and have had these six healthy children. I've had a checkup recently. X rays show that my heart is not enlarged, and my ECG's are normal, too.

"I can't understand why so many people with heart disease worry about it so much. As in everything else in life, you have to have faith."

I told her that some day I would repeat her interesting and uplifting story in print. And so I have done, to bring hope to any reader who is greatly concerned about having a child because she has a murmur due to rheumatic heart disease.

I keep reminding people that all heart disease is not cut out of one pattern. It varies. One patient may be seriously ill with rheumatic heart disease while ten others live normal and long lives.

16.

CONGENITAL
HEART DISEASE

Simply put, congenital heart disease means that heart damage has occurred in the fetus before it is born as a full-grown baby. In many cases the cause is unknown. In others, we think we can trace it to the mother having had German measles during the first few months after conception, or having taken some harmful drug, or having been exposed to X rays during this vital period in the development of the baby.

Some congenital hearts are so deformed that the baby is not alive at birth. In most, however, there is damage ranging from minimal to serious, but susceptible to operative repair. Not too many years ago we were unable to make any repairs. With the remarkable advances in cardiac surgery, however, thousands of potential congenital heart invalids have been transformed into normal human beings.

Although surgical experience is essential for good results, diagnosis still remains an important part of the entire procedure. The significant question that must be answered is this: Is it or isn't it congenital heart disease? Is it only, for example, a harmless functional murmur?

Here is a typical letter I received some time ago from a frustrated parent:

> Our young son has a heart murmur. He has been to a number of doctors. There is a difference of opinion. Some say he has only what they call a functional murmur and have advised us to forget it. They told him to play tennis and football and to behave like any other normal youngster.
>
> But after an examination by one of the best heart specialists at a large, well-known medical school in our city, we were told that he is not so sure it is functional. He thinks it is possible that our boy may have congenital heart disease—a small opening between the left and right sides of the heart. It is important, he says, to do a heart catheterization. This will tell the true story. Will you explain what is meant by this procedure? Is it dangerous?

My reply to this justifiably worried mother went as follows:

> I'll answer your second question first. Any surgical procedure has an element of danger, whether it is minor or major surgery. But the experience with this process in thousands of patients indicates that complications are rare, even though it seems to be a very serious procedure.
>
> Heart catheterizations means just that—inserting a catheter (a long hollow tube which is quite flexible) directly into the heart itself. A small incision is made in an arm vein; the long, soft, pliable catheter is gently pushed up the vein until it enters the heart cavity. The operator helps its guidance by fluoroscope.
>
> By examining blood specimens and by taking pressures in the heart cavity, the diagnostician can determine whether or not there is actual damage to the heart

208

—either to its valves or muscles or to the septum (the wall dividing left heart from right).

In expert hands the heart catheterization takes about an hour and is relatively painless. In view of your son's problem you deserve to know the actual truth about his heart. Otherwise, he will go through life not knowing whether to live like a semi-invalid or to engage in all normal activities. Since there is a difference of medical opinion, and an experienced cardiologist advises the examination, it is logical to follow his advice.

Earlier in this book I indicated how important it is to know whether a patient has organic heart disease or imaginary heart trouble. This is a certain way in which to make the distinction. Besides, if it is congenital heart disease, the patient can look forward to a successful surgical result and a lifetime of normal activity.

The wonders of modern heart surgery augur well for the patient who is otherwise doomed to slow, steady deterioration caused by increasing heart failure due to congenital heart disease—or to many other types of apparently hopeless heart disease.

PART IV

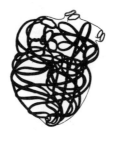

LIVE HAPPILY
A LONG TIME AFTER

17.

HOW TO BE LESS ANXIOUS
ABOUT REAL HEART DISEASE

*If you really are afflicted with heart disease it is not un-
likely that you, too, have an overlay of anxiety about
your heart. You might ask, "Who has a better right to
be concerned—you or the patient with imaginery heart
trouble?"*

*But anxiety knows no bounds. It does not make any
effort to distinguish between real and imaginary trouble. It
disturbs the equanimity of the man who has had a coronary
attack as it does the healthy man who has been frightened
by heart skips.*

*In this section I'll make some practical suggestions for
those of you who have indisputable evidence of actual
heart disease. If you are one of the many who have lost faith
in this inherently powerful bundle of muscle, I'll try to
show you that* your heart is stronger than you think.

I was tempted to call this chapter "The Corpse that
Came to Life." But I had a meeting with myself and
voted *no*.

My reasons? This is not a collection of detective stories. But more important, life and death are dramatic
enough; it is not necessary to apply artificial stimulus to

create interest in what is already of tremendous importance to all of us. Anyone who has been the leading character in a heart attack does not need to have his memory jogged into recalling the pain and anxiety that were interwoven to highlight that dramatic experience.

Yet, "The Corpse That Came to Life" is not an exaggerated and phony title. It is based on the actual case history of a patient I treated years ago. In more than twenty-five years of practice, his was the severest attack of coronary thrombosis I have ever observed personally, or read about, who recovered.

For months, I had been treating a fifty-year-old benign, kindly man. He was a successful insurance broker who spoke so softly one had to lean forward to hear him distinctly. I guess he was successful because he was a soft-sell rather than a hard-sell salesman. His character was an example that the sure-fire formula for success is what I call "ability plus likability."

He came to me for checkups about once a month. I had made the diagnosis of angina pectoris about a year previously. He had some changes in his electrocardiograms and especially complained of occasional pains in his chest when he walked against the wind on a cold day. He would stop, put a nitroglycerine tablet under his tongue, and within minutes be on his way again. He had been experiencing an average of a half-dozen attacks daily.

This day of his appointment there were no unusual findings. ECG's showed no change from previous heart tracings. His attacks were not more frequent. We chatted a while before he was about to leave. I recall I reassured him, but warned against any sudden, heavy exertion.

He smiled, his mild blue eyes crinkling in his round, moon-like face, and said, "I try to be a good patient."

214

Later I learned that he had pushed and half-carried four heavily laden trash barrels from his backyard to the front sidewalk that very evening because his son, whose job it was, had not expected to be home until later that night.

About 11:30 P.M. his son telephoned in a state of near panic. "Doctor, please come right over. My dad is having terrible chest pains. I am very worried about him. He looks as if he's dying."

When I reached the broker's home about twenty minutes later, he was covered with a heavy layer of sweat. His face was ashen. His eyeballs rolled upward. His hands clutched at his chest. He moaned and twisted.

I listened to his heart and could barely hear it. After injecting a large dose of morphine, I took his blood pressure. It had fallen from 160 (while in the office that afternoon) to 80 systolic.

The family stood nearby: wife, son and daughter. Their faces mirrored their anxiety. In fact, the wife was close to tears and her lips kept moving soundlessly. Finally the son blurted out the question preying on all their minds.

"Is he going to be all right, Doctor?"

I told them he was having an attack of coronary thrombosis. It was not necessary for me to spell out the seriousness of the situation. No medical training was necessary to realize that the prognosis was bad. Here, for all to see, was a critically ill man.

I continued to sit by his bedside, administering the routine treatment. By 1 A.M. his blood pressure had fallen to 40 systolic. He groaned less and moved less. The family looked pleadingly at me and I tried not to avoid meeting their imploring eyes. In fact, I did my best not to act as if I were dealing with a hopelessly dying man.

215

At 2 A.M. his blood pressure had slipped to zero. Nor could I hear his heart beats. Except for an almost imperceptible movement of his chest, he seemed already a corpse.

Yet, something happened that I cannot explain to this day. Certainly, it was not because of any dramatic new treatment I had instituted, but a few pulse beats began to come through. Then more and more, irregularly, it is true, but they fluttered by. Finally, at 5 A.M. his blood pressure had climbed back to 60.

From then on, for at least a week, we were all skating on thin ice. Although not practically dead my patient was not completely alive either.

But I won't take you through the following weeks and months in detail. The main point I wish to make is that he survived.

I reported his case history to the Hartford Medical Society on or about the first anniversary of his attack as an example of how a critically ill coronary patient can recover and live for a year in the face of a hopeless prognosis.

I recall that I tried to impress the members that the old saying "While there's life there's hope" is not as outdated as it seems. Little did I realize at the time that my full optimism about coronary cases had not yet been realized.

Years later I had occasion to make another report—including this patient's history—to the *Annals of Internal Medicine,* the official publication of the American College of Physicians. This apparent corpse had survived his coronary attack for twenty years! He lived until the age of seventy and died of cancer—not of his heart ailment. (Each year of those twenty years he used to bring me

216

fresh tomatoes from his garden in thankfulness and in memory of the anniversary of his heart attack.)

I present this case history as only one example to prove that suffering a heart attack does not invariably mean one's life is over. There have been reports in medical literature of patients living a quarter of a century after an attack—or after several attacks.

Today we are much more optimistic about the average life expectancy of one who has had a heart attack than we would have been ten or twenty years ago. The younger you are, the longer your future life expectancy. One-third of coronary attack patients will be able to return to a full schedule of work after their convalescence. Another third will have to slow down a bit. The final third will have to take it much easier. The chances of becoming a bedridden invalid are only about one in twenty.

Over the years coronary patients have asked me thousands of questions regarding themselves and the disease. From the long list of answers I have evolved a formula for telling patients, in simple language, what they ought to know to prevent and manage coronary disease.

In the following few pages, you will find the distillate of what I consider the necessary common-sense procedure people should follow if they hope to neutralize the inroads coronary disease has been making during the past half-century.

If what I say here becomes second nature to you in planning your way of life, you will be less likely to become a victim of a coronary attack. And if you suffer an attack, you will be more likely to survive and return to a normal program of daily living.

Here are some of the questions as I have heard them, and some of the answers as I have given them:

217

Is coronary disease on the increase?

This is debatable. Perhaps there seems to be more coronary disease around because of better diagnosis and more up-to-date statistics, and the population explosion.

What's the difference between angina pectoris and coronary thrombosis?

In the former there usually has been a gradual narrowing of one or both coronary arteries; in the latter, closure is most often complete and sudden.

Is overweight really harmful?

Insurance company statisticians will tell you that the person who is fifty pounds overweight has a greater than 50 percent likelihood of dying in the coming year than his normal-weight neighbor.

Is it safe to fly?

Generally speaking, if you are well enough to walk you are well enough to fly.

Shall I tell my wife?

Without exception she should be "the first to know." Many a wife has prolonged the life of her husband for many years because she was taken into the doctor's confidence. And many a man has died prematurely solely "because his wife didn't know."

Must I take a vacation every year?

Many people look upon vacations as a luxury they cannot afford. On the contrary, they are a *necessity* that we cannot do without. We need periodic "recharging." Otherwise, we go through life like a rundown battery.

What is a good modern heart examination?

It consists of much more than a stethoscope survey: X rays, electrocardiograms, and laboratory tests.

Do you advise early retirement?

This is an individual problem. A satisfactory retirement requires years of psychological, as well as economic, preparation. Some men are so constituted physically and emotionally that they are better advised to continue working into their seventies; others are wiser if they retire during their fifties.

How can one avoid being tense in this modern world?

It is possible to learn how to relax. But it takes practice. People give up too soon. As in learning to play the violin or piano, you must persevere until you have learned how to keep your cool.

How about sex relations?

This, too, depends upon one's glands, emotional make-up, and the condition of the circulation. Do not be shy about discussing this important question with your doctor. His answer may relieve you of much physical and emotional distress.

How about work? When? How much?

Before your attack of thrombosis or your symptoms of angina, you may have been fully suited to your work. However, after the diagnosis has been made, you would be well advised to review the work situation with your doctor. You may now be a square peg in a round hole. A change, therefore, may be in order.

219

What about heart operations?

During the last twenty-five years there have been greater advances in heart management than in the 2,500 years preceding. The modern heart operation, transplant or otherwise, is only one example of this progress. In indicated cases, an operation can be helpful to the coronary patient.

Can I continue smoking?

It's a long story. If there is any doubt at all—in your mind or in your doctor's—stop entirely! I have known few patients who were able to "cut down" satisfactorily.

How about a nip of alcohol?

I have advised most patients over forty—whether they had coronary trouble or not—to take an ounce or two of liquor before dinner every night. It helps cut the rope of the day's tension and makes for relaxed eating and pleasant relationships at the table. (And over the years, I have never observed such patients turn into chronic alcoholics.)

Is it necessary for every thrombosis patient to have "blood thinners"?

No. Some patients need to take heparin and dicumarol from the very beginning, and continue to take it for months and years. Others get along very well without it. *Who's who* and *which is which* depends entirely upon the experience of the attending physician.

Are low-cholesterol diets important for the coronary patient?

They are. Especially for those individuals with a history of a recent attack or for those (not having had an attack)

220

who have high cholesterol levels in their blood. However, we do not have the entire answer to the cholesterol problem. That is why some doctors put their patients on strict low cholesterol foods; others are more lenient. They say, "Just cut down on fats and fried foods. We don't know enough about the cholesterol mystery to be more specific than that."

Have I the right to call in a consultant?

By all means do. It's worth it for peace of mind. Your doctor shouldn't object.

Is bed rest as necessary as it used to be?

During an attack of coronary thrombosis patients in the past were kept in bed for many weeks and months —sometimes three or four months. Now we keep them in bed three to six weeks. In fact, some cardiologists allow their patients to sit up in a chair within a day or two after the attack. Most doctors, however, believe in taking the middle-of-the-road policy of conservatism.

How much nitroglycerine can I take?

Most patients are "scared" of the name nitroglycerine. They associate it with dynamite and "blowing to bits." Therefore, many suffer unnecessarily. They should take it more often. If necessary, there's no harm in taking one or two dozen tablets a day.

Do electrocardiograms always tell the true story?

Heart tracings are invaluable. Nevertheless, they are only one part of our weapons used to manage coronary disease. Sometimes the electrocardiogram will tell us all we want to know. Most often, we are not content without

221

the help of a complete history, physical examination, and laboratory tests.

Does climate make any difference?

Many patients have increased their heart power simply by moving to a warm and equable climate. On the contrary, there are many others who seem unmindful of the weather. However, I advise coronary patients to follow the sun!

How can a wife help her husband after a coronary attack?

The wife is really the doctor's first assistant. She is often the only means for seeing that the doctor's orders are carried out. That helps save lives.

What is atherosclerosis?

The arteries become hard and brittle. They lose their youthful elasticity. This is due to the laying down between the inner arterial coat, layers of cholesterol and lime salts that later interfere with the free flow of blood through the arteries. This is the most common cause of loss of heart power.

Is exercise dangerous?

Without any equivocation I say it is. You hear it said that exercise never hurt the healthy heart. True! But what forty-year-old heart (or over) is healthy compared with a healthy teen-aged heart? Yet many middle-aged athletes insist upon proving to others and to themselves that the "old boy is just as good as he used to be." That's when coronary patients (potential and real) get into serious trouble. They call on heart power they haven't got.

Are visitors sometimes a serious problem?

Many patients in recent coronary attacks have had seri-

222

ous relapses because they have been tired out by tactless visitors. No sign is more important for the coronary patient than the *No Visitors* sign which so many people ignore.

Does a patient with diabetes have to be especially careful?

His diet should be low in cholesterol foods because such patients have a tendency to have high blood-cholesterol levels. And the diabetic should be especially careful not to take too large a dose of insulin. In lowering the blood sugar suddenly he may interfere with the nourishment in the coronary arteries.

Is indigestion an important symptom?

"Acute indigestion" was the term used years ago in headlines describing what we learned later to be attacks of coronary thrombosis. We are always suspicious of a person over forty (especially a male) who complains of severe indigestion—or any kind of indigestion that "hangs on" longer than usual. In such cases, taking serial electrocardiograms and blood-enzyme tests are a necessity. Otherwise, the diagnosis is easily missed.

Can you have a bad heart even though the electrocardiogram is normal?

Yes.

Just what is the value of periodic heart checkups?

Putting out a match flame is easy; trying to control a conflagration is something else again. The same is true for heart disease. The patient has a better chance if the problem is discovered early so that appropriate corrective measures can be taken.

The foregoing are among the more frequent questions

223

that prick the anxious minds of the coronary patient and his family. Other questions and their answers are intrinsic to the various aspects of organic heart disease and imaginary heart disease discussed in earlier chapters in this book.

In any event, our job as doctors is to tell you what road to take—and how to drive your machine. We can only make the diagnosis and prescribe the treatment. The *living* of your life is entirely up to *you*. Your heart is in your own hands!

Therefore, take the following advice and make it part of your way of life:

Practical Pointers for Coronary Patients

1. Never overeat.
2. Don't exert yourself immediately after a meal; rest at least one-half hour.
3. When you leave your house on a cold day, cover your mouth and nose with handkerchief or scarf until you get accustomed to the cold.
4. If you can prevent it, never walk uphill against a brisk wind on a cold day.
5. Try taking a nitroglycerine pill *before* any exertion similar to one that brought on the pain previously.
6. Never shovel snow.
7. Never "run" after anything.
8. If you get a flat tire at midnight on a lonely country road, don't change it. If you can't get help, determine to sleep right where you are until morning.
9. Don't smoke or remain for any length of time in a smoke-filled room.
10. Try to control your emotions. A fit of temper is

worse than running upstairs. It has killed many an anginal patient.

11. Simply because the electrocardiogram was normal don't disbelieve the diagnosis of angina your doctor has made.

12. If your present job is too much for you—either physically or emotionally—change it. If you determine to stick it out, you may "get stuck."

13. Take frequent rest periods. Learn how to take naps "at the drop of a hat."

14. Don't let the hands of the clock choke you as you rush from appointment to appointment. Get up a half-hour earlier. Leave free periods on your calendar. Otherwise, you will be crowding too much work into twenty-four hours.

15. Don't fill up on "fat" snacks before bedtime. Too much fat overloading the bloodstream may predispose to a coronary thrombosis attack.

16. The only exercise you need is moderate walking. Try to increase the distance gradually—and within your pain limits. This kind of exercise often helps build collateral (new) circulation in the coronary branches.

17. If caught in an air terminal or railway station with two heavy bags and no porter, don't risk the heart strain of carrying them a few hundred yards to a taxi.

18. In stair climbing "level out steps" by resting on every other step to the count of five.

19. You may have a daily ration of two or three ounces of scotch, rye, bourbon, or brandy. It may help cut down on nitroglycerine needs. But never drink before driving.

20. See your doctor periodically even though you feel well.

21. Don't worry about your illness. Optimistic patients do best.

22. Do as the doctor says—not as he does.

23. Here's a simple way to test your coronary arteries. Try to walk 120 steps in 60 seconds (but don't force it). If you can do so without pain under your chest (especially on a cold day, and walking up a slope after a meal) chances are your coronaries are doing a serviceable job.

24. Don't strain when constipated if you can help it. If there's not a choice, be sure that you keep your mouth open. (If you strain against a closed mouth, it puts a heavy burden on your heart). Try to overcome constipation by taking mineral oil and milk of magnesia occasionally.

25. If you are confined to bed by a cold or for some other reason, don't lie immobile too long. That favors getting a thrombus (clot) in your heart or lungs. Every few hours, flex the muscles of your arms, feet, and legs. Bend your legs on your thighs. This will help prevent stagnation of blood and resultant complications.

27. Be sure to check with your doctor if anginal pains come more frequently and after less effort. That may be a warning that a thrombosis is on the way.

28. Remember that your heart and your life are in your own hands. Constant good care is the secret of longevity and good health. Commit these wise words of Dr. Lawrason Brown to memory and say them once a day: "After all, the most important thing is to be able to control one's self. Unless a patient can say 'no' when the occasion arises, his chances for getting well are very slight. He can tear down in one day or in an hour what it has taken many months to build up. A man often dies on account of his disposition rather than on account of his disease."

29. When warned against high cholesterol, don't fill

226

up on ice cream, fatty meats, fried foods, eggs, cream, or pastry.

30. Don't put off a needed vacation.
31. Don't stay fat! You invite diabetes, high blood pressure, coronary disease, kidney disease, or stroke.
32. Don't be overly ambitious; learn how to sit in the back row—and *enjoy* it!
33. Learn to control your emotions. Don't fly into a rage or nurse chronic resentment.
34. Don't be fatalistic and say, "There's nothing anybody can do for heart trouble; when your number's up, it's up!"
35. Remember that middle-aged arteries are inelastic. Don't overexercise.
36. Don't try to prove to yourself that you are as good as you used to be. Don't play seventy-two holes of golf on a weekend, or take on a teenager for five sets of singles in tennis, or indulge too vigorously in calisthenics.
37. If you are the wife of a coronary patient, continue nagging him to take good care of himself. It's better to be called a nagger of a live husband than it is to become a widow.
38. Don't live in tension. Don't try to pile twenty-eight hours of work into a twenty-four-hour day.
39. Learn how to take an afternoon and evening nap.
40. Don't let the telephone bedevil you.
41. Don't allow the hands of the clock to choke you into submission.
42. Don't eat a stale cheese sandwich and drink a glass of warm milk off your desk top. Take the time to enjoy an adequate and sensible lunch in congenial surroundings.
43. Don't try to diagnose or treat yourself.

227

44. Sexual activity? Don't let prudery deter you from obtaining your physician's advice in this area.

Knowing these things should help remove many layers of anxiety from your mind. It is the vague and the unknown that impose such a daily strain on our lives.

EPILOGUE

If you are heart-sick (real or imaginary) where does hope begin? Where does it end?

The answers can be found only in yourself, your doctor—and your family's understanding. Medicine and surgery are not the end-all, the cure-all. Even though your doctor has done a good job, you must have faith in his directives and capabilities. Complete empathy on his part and faith on your part are the natural ingredients for forming the base of mutual understanding and cooperation that can bring you health, happiness, and peace of mind.

For example, suppose you have had a serious attack of coronary thrombosis. After many weeks of care and rest, your physician says you are now able to return to work. Most patients are happy to comply. They have faith in what their doctor says. Yet, some people question the recommendations of their physicians.

In my own practice I have known such persons. Because of anxiety—nurtured by faithlessness and hopelessness—they take themselves out of the mainstream of life. They give up business. They stop playing golf. They abandon their former way of life and exist as semi-invalids. All because they do not believe their doctor implicitly.

However, as I said earlier, we doctors should remember that the patient's faith in us does not grow on barren soil. Although it is true that some patients develop complete belief in their physician as soon as they see his shingle, white coat, or stethoscope, most individuals need personal, sympathetic care by their doctor before they can commit themselves wholeheartedly to his guidance and specific ministrations.

Not only must your doctor be a well-trained medical man to inspire faith; he must be a human being with empathy, understanding, kindness, patience, a sense of humor, and confidence in himself, and have an unrestrained urge to help his patient.

(Believe it or not, you will have to take my word that the majority of physicians are like this when not handcuffed by lack of time. It pays to search for such a one until you find him.)

Millions in the United States continue to live in fear because of imaginary heart trouble. For them there is no longer any joy. They suffer the agony and torture known only to those who live in the shadow of what they believe is imminent doom.

Peace of mind and peace of soul—you can have neither without peace of heart.

It is evident that you must not *guess* that you have heart disease. Instead, you should summon the courage to find out. Why live a half a life when you can live a whole one?

All this presupposes that both you and your doctor have a job to do. He will not "laugh off" your fears and dismiss you with a perfunctory "forget it." After examining you with all the diagnostic equipment at his command—a full physical checkup, fluoroscopic and X-ray surveys, electrocardiograms, and the indicated laboratory tests—he will tell you the truth about your condition.

Either you have heart disease or you do not. There is no indeterminate buffer zone.

If the diagnosis is actual heart disease, you can be thankful that he discovered it early. Your doctor will prescribe medicine and a new way of life that will prolong your years.

If the diagnosis is imaginary heart trouble (and that is what three out of four persons actually have who think they are saddled with heart disease) he will give you reassurance and the necessary medications to overcome your discomforts and fears.

If you are "heart-scared" do something about it now. Your need is not to wonder, but to know. Make an appointment with an able physician. He will help you combat your chronic anxiety.

But the crux of it all is this. Having been told your heart is normal—by means of a thorough medical and laboratory evaluation—try to discard whatever fears you may have when your doctor hands down a verdict of "heart not guilty." Accept it with relief. Believe him.

Otherwise, you will soon be riding the crowded medical merry-go-round, going from doctor to doctor, feeling worse and worse as you try to find one whom you can bring yourself to believe. This constant rejection of carefully assembled medical facts is the green arrow that leads inevitably to the psychiatrist's couch.

Your prime contribution as a patient is to believe in the doctor you consult. You must assume that he is eager to help and that he will be sincere and honest in passing along his findings to you.

In conclusion, let me say that my purpose in writing

231

this book has not been so much to bring you specific information as to instill faith in yourself and the durability of your heart. By narrating a number of case histories taken out of my personal medical files and from letters written by readers o fmy nationally syndicated newspaper column, I have revealed the intimate experiences of men and women who suffered unreasonably and often needlessly from heart trouble. I want to save you from that ingrained but often unexpressed fear that people go around suddenly dropping dead.

Whether you have real heart disease or imaginary heart trouble, I hope in reading what I have had to say that you have come to share my sincere conviction that your heart is stronger than you think, so that you may enjoy life without the added burden of daily anxiety.

Your heart is in your own hands.

Henry D. Thoreau said, "It takes two to speak truth— one to speak and another to hear."

I have spoken. Have you heard?

232

INDEX